Wudang Qigong

Second Edition

China's

Wudang Mountain

Daoist Breath Exercises

by Yuzeng Liu

Translated by Yuzeng Liu and Terri Morgan

First Edition

Chinese portion of this text is excerpted from Wudang Qigong

Original translation of the excerpted text

Photographs

First Edition Published in 1999
ISBN 0-9672889-0-8

Second Edition

New and revised translation

Second Edition Published in 2023
ISBN-13: 978-0-9672889-8-7
ISBN-10: 0-9672889-8-3

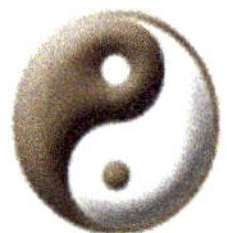

Wudang Research Association

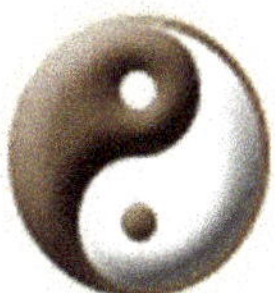

Now this book "Wudang Daoist Breath Exercises" is offered as a tribute and is given to everyone in the whole world who loves qigong and martial arts, and to weave goodwill among all. May everyone have a smooth, peaceful, and long life.

Table of Contents

Forward to the Second Edition

The Wudang Research Association (International Wudang Internal Martial Arts Research Association) was founded in 1996 by Terri Morgan and Liu Yuzeng to translate and publish his books and essays on Wudang Internal Arts and other topics. Our first print publication was the first edition of this book in 1999.

By 1996, Professor Liu was very well-known in China. In addition to Wudang Arts, Liu Yuzeng is a highly respected teacher of Shaolin Arts and is known as Shi De Yu. His teacher was Shi Su Xi. He wrote several sections in the four-volume Encyclopedia of Shaolin Martial Arts. He had published several books and hundreds of articles, including a book on Wudang Qigong. He wanted to have his books translated to English and published in the US.

We looked at his book on Wudang Qigong first. He had been teaching classes. Students wanted something to reference. But the material was going to be difficult to translate. He had included sections from the Classics (Laozi, Kongzi, and others with commentary). The Chinese Classics are difficult to understand anyway. That's why he included commentary. Back then, I wasn't ready to attempt a translation of the Classics. But I could translate the movements. I was learning the Traditional Chinese Medicine (TCM) concepts and the internal workmanship. I could translate that. So he reviewed what he had, took out the references to the Classics, and we began creating a new book.

It took me about two years to translate and edit. I was careful. I paid attention to the words and what I understood about practice. So many times what was literal was not the correct meaning. Other times, what was common language was wrong for qigong practice. Even so, I knew there would be a few things I would miss or that wouldn't be quite what they should.

Wudang Qigong

With this second edition, I have reviewed my original translation and made a few changes. My Chinese has gotten better. I have corrected more than a few mistakes. I've tried to make the instructions a little easier to read while still keeping as close to the original as possible. That also means that where there are commas in the original, there are commas that maybe should be periods in the translation. The instructions for performing the exercises are not separate. Each segment is connected – the same as the exercises should be.

I've adjusted the formatting. We intended that first edition to be printed and used as a reference in class. As we considered how to set it up, we decided on having the Chinese and English on facing pages to use a teaching tool. Back then, ebooks were very limited. Today, ebooks are common and print may be harder to find. This edition keeps the Chinese and English in one book but separates them for continuous viewing as an ebook. The new printed version uses this layout, too.

The photos of Professor Liu included in this edition were taken in 2006 in Zhengzhou, Henan.

It is now 2023. Many things have happened in the 30 years since I met Professor Liu at People's Park in Zhengzhou in January 1991 during Spring Festival. He was teaching Xingyi class that cold winter morning. I stopped to watch. He invited me to learn.

It is my hope that this book will preserve traditional Wudang Qigong, Professor Liu's teachings, and my own contributions as a student, translator, and teacher.

- Terri Morgan
7/23/2023

Preface

Because the source of China's Wudang Mountain Daoist Breath Exercises is in the Wudang Mountains,[1] this resulted in its name. The Wudang Mountains are also called the Shen Shang Mountains and the Tai He Mountains; they are one of the places in China sacred to Daoists. It is always said "Since ancient times unrivaled superb scenery, under Heaven the first immortal mountains;" and "In the North Shaolin has great importance;" and "In the South Wudang is revered."

Wudang Qigong supports the human body by acting as "fire in the cauldron;" thus refining and cultivating the energy, inner breath, and spirit inside the body; refining the inner center. Use the intention to circulate the inner breath then use the inner breath to urge the body, collect the spirit, clear the mind, embrace emptiness and hold onto the one. A person who practices can then dispel disease, strengthen the body, prolong the years, and increase the life span. By circulating the inner breath using the five elements and the eight methods it is possible to resist the unhealthy influences that cause disease and guard against their savagery. Indeed, internally it can preserve one's health, externally it can dispel evil, inside and outside are both cultivated using these distinct and unique methods for practicing inner breath exercises.

According to legend, during the Eastern Han dynasty Yin Changsheng, during the Jin dynasty Xie Yun, during the Tang dynasty Liu Dongbin, during the Ming dynasty Zhang Sanfeng, all cultivated and refined themselves in these mountains.[2] "Zhang

---

[1] The Wudang Mountains lie along the northwest border of Hubei province in Jun County. In the Han dynasty, the name of the mountains was Wudang Xian and they were part of Nan Yang prefecture.

[2] See The Dictionary of Religion, p. 625, notes on "Wudang Mountain."

Sanfeng was good at opening the valley pathway"[3] and was widely acclaimed and welcomed by people at that time as a Daoist Scholar.[4]

Now, we in presenting this book, compiled and written based on materials provided by Master Wang Xixiao[5] for this family of Wudang Qigong. These materials include his personal instruction in Wudang Qigong, his secret Qigong book and relevant Daoist methods for cultivating character and refining breath which have been put in order and compiled. This book is dedicated to all Wudang Qigong enthusiasts. Because Wudang Breath Exercises has many methods, it is difficult to include all of them. I sincerely ask Qigong masters both in China and overseas to explore, arrange, and supplement thereby enabling another step toward perfection.

During the course of compiling this book, to the Wudang Mountain Wudang Boxing Research Association, Secretary General Huang Xuewen who paid close attention and gave support, as equally did the Henan Police Upper Division

---

[3] "辟谷" (Pì Gǔ) is a concept commonly found in traditional Chinese medicine and Daoist culture. Literally translated, it means "opening up the valley pathway." In this context, "辟谷" refers to a special dietary and lifestyle practice aimed at achieving body purification, health maintenance, and spiritual cultivation through controlled eating and, in some cases, abstaining from solid foods.

[4] See The History of Daoism, p. 262.

[5] Wang Xixiao 王希孝 Shifu (1893-1986): was from Mengjin county near Luoyang in Henan. When he was small he studied taijiquan with a fifth generation descendant of venerated teacher Wang Zongyue. Later, obeying his teacher's instruction he went to the Wudang Mountains and became a disciple of Daoist Master Li Heqi. After Liberation (1949), he returned to his hometown and became a close friend of my respected grandfather Liu Wenzhou. Afterward, in Zhengzhou City's People's Park he established a place to instruct students.

Academy, Henan Sports Publications Society, Henan Province Health First Qigong Federation, Zhengzhou City Martial and Wudang Boxing Research Association. To all the good friends and disciples who gave their energetic assistance, I sincerely extend my thanks. In the course of translating this book, I received wholehearted and dedicated assistance from the US International Wudang Internal Martial Arts Research Association. For this I am extremely grateful.

Yuzeng Liu
June 28, 1999

Wudang Qigong

China's
Wudang Mountain
Daoist Breath Exercises

Section 1: Wudang Qigong: Introduction

Daoist Qigong has eighteen sets of practice exercises and methods: Extreme Emptiness, Pushing the Mountain, Wild Goose Flying, Crane Bending, Supporting Heaven, Both Appear, Four Directions, Ward Off and Pull Down, Pipa, Shaking Tail Feathers, Offering Fruit, Facing the Sun, Stirring the Grass, Dragon and Tiger, Coiling Snake, Spitting a Core, Climbing a Tree, and Bowing To The Top. The practice of Daoist Qigong is primarily one person practice, with the guidance of a teacher, paying attention to respiration, breath circulation, breath distribution, embryonic (pre-birth) breathing, etc. and can be practiced and studied sitting, lying down, and moving.

The first step is to move the inner breath in the small heavenly circle. This is also known as the first gate and is called refining the energy and transforming the breath. Together energy, breath, and spirit become spirit breath. The second step is to move the inner breath in the large heavenly circle. This is known as the middle gate and is called refining the breath and transforming the spirit. Together spirit and breath become spirit. The third step is combining ten thousand things into an integral whole, this is known as refining the spirit and returning to emptiness,[6] clearing the mind reveals the nature, strengthens the body, and prolongs the years.

Energy, inner breath, spirit, refer to inherent aspects of the human body, original essence, original breath, original spirit. Among these, energy is the foundation, breath is the impetus, and spirit is the master. By harnessing the spirit, inner breath can be controlled; by refining the spirit, energy is cultivated. In the human body, when the energy is consolidated, then the inner breath will be sufficient. When the spirit is sufficient, then vigor will be abundant and the body and mind will be healthy. Conversely, if the energy is depleted, the breath will be exhausted, and when the breath is exhausted, then the spirit diminishes. Consequently, in the process of refining and cultivating, it is essential to constantly focus on nurturing and preserving vitality, regulating inner breath, and conserving the spirit. When the energy is complete, the breath will be strong. When the breath is strong, the spirit will flourish. A flourishing spirit leads to a healthy body free from disease.

Laozi's Dao Te Jing in the third chapter says "Empty the mind, fill the belly. Weaken the ambition, strengthen the bones."[7] So then, these are the maxims for practicing China's

---

[6] 无极 wu ji - empty of everything, receptive to everything

[7] 虚 xu - Hsu, vacuous. "A Daoist term often used by Neo-Confucianists also. As a description of a state of mind, it means absolute peacefulness and purity of mind and freedom from worry and selfish desires and not to be disturbed by incoming impressions or to allow what is already in the mind to disturb what is coming into the mind. Hsu-shih means unreality and reality, but hsu also means profound and deep continuum in which there is no obstruction." in Chan, Wing Tsit. A Source Book on Chinese Philosophy, Princeton: Princeton U. Press, 1973, p. 788.

Wing Tsit Chan translates this passage as ... keeps their hearts vacuous (虚 xu), fills their bellies, weakens their ambitions, and strengthens their bones... ibid, p. 141.

Daoist Qigong. When learning to practice, one must understand it thoroughly and become proficient in it. If you haven't mastered one method of practicing Daoist qigong, temporarily don't practice other training methods. If you are unfamiliar with a specific movement, concentrate on that posture before studying or practicing other postures. Avoid aiming too high too soon, instead approach practice with humility and perseverance, simultaneously nurturing both inside and outside. Step by step achieve a state where the abdomen is relaxed and the inner breath rises naturally, directly nurturing without harm. Fill the Dan Tian with the inner breath and allow it to circulate unimpeded and unobstructed, let the breath and the strength be sent out from the spine, according to that which the mind desires. Be dedicated and realistic. Practice carefully and maintain it so it will be lasting. Follow the guidelines for each movement, cultivate the inner breath to nurture the body, refine the mind to nourish the spirit in order to achieve emptiness, tranquility, and long life.

Robert Blakney translates this passage as "... to empty people's hearts and minds, to fill their bellies, weaken their ambition, give them sturdy frames and always so..... The explanation given in the paraphrase is that this means "... stilling individual appetites and ambitions among the people,..., so that the virtue of the Way may show in all." Blakney, Robert B. The Way of Life Tao Tzu Tao Te Ching: A New Translation by R. B. Blakney, New York: New American Library, 1955. p. 55.

Section 2: Wudang Qigong: Subtle Effects

Chinese Daoist Qigong, known in ancient times as "Dao Yin," "Tu Na," "Lian Qi," "Lian Dan," "Zuo Guan," "Bi Gu," or simply referred to as "Nei Gong" (inner cultivation), has a long history of widespread circulation among the people. In 1973 (CE) at Changsha,[8] the "Dao Yin Tu" painting on silk was unearthed from the Western Han dynasty tombs at Mawangdui[9] with 44 distinct postures and gestures showing movements for refining the breath. The famous ancient medical doctor Hua Tuo[10] taught the movements of the Five Animal Frolics to Wu Jin to promote healthy bodies, dispel disease, and prolong life.[11] Zhuang Zi said: "Exhaling the old and receiving the new is like the stretching of a bear or the extending of a bird's neck. Those who practice "Dao Yin" also cultivate their outer form." Regular practice of China's Daoist Qigong methods, cultivating the inner breath, results in improved digestion, open blood vessels, helps prevent disease, and for people it is also the key to not deteriorating. As centuries of practice have shown, practicing Daoist Qigong plays an important role in preventing disease, treatment of disease, physical well-being, and longevity.

---

[8] Changsha, Hunan Province. "The site of Changsha has been inhabited for 3000 years. By the Warring States Period (770-221 BCE) a large town had grown up." China: A Travel Survival Kit. Berkeley, CA: Lonely Planet, May 1988, p. 301.

[9] The Hunan Provincial Museum is on Dongfeng Lu (in Changsha)... two buildings are devoted to the 2100 year old Western Han tombs at Mawangdui....Large quantities of silk garments and fabrics were found in the tomb...." ibid. p. 302.

[10] 华佗 Hua Tuo (Han dynasty)

[11] "Hua Tuo,... created the Five Animal Frolics, based on the movements of cranes, bears, deer, monkeys, and tigers." Deng, Mingdao. The Scholar Warrior. HarperCollins: New York, 1990, p. 39.

Part 1: Effects on the Respiratory System

The functions of the respiratory system are to breathe in thus receiving oxygen from the outside world and to discharge carbon dioxide from inside the body, thus guaranteeing the normal functioning of the body's metabolic processes. When practicing Wudang Qigong, special respiration patterns are employed, such as inverse (or reverse) style breathing, throat breathing, Dan Tian breathing, and so on, in order to increase activity in the five internal organs and six bowels,[12] and because it consumes a large quantity of energy, this prompts the respiratory organs to double their work, so breathing in takes in a greater amount of oxygen (this is also clear breath) at the same time discharging a greater amount of carbon dioxide (this is also dirty breath); thereby both receive a very good workout. Particularly notable is the practice of "sinking the breath to the Dan Tian" a breathing method that uses the movement of the diaphragm and which has shown notable effects in medical care and nationwide fitness programs.

The principle manifestations of improvement in respiratory system functions are in the activity of the outer wall of the chest and in the increased capacity of the lungs. Typically, when breathing in deeply, the span of the chest compared with breathing out is 7-9 centimeters greater and the amount the lungs move is 3500 milliliters more or less. But in a person who practices Wudang Qigong regularly, the chest expansion can reach 9-18 centimeters and the frequency of respiration can be reduced. An ordinary person breathes in and out 15-20 times each minute, but in a person who regularly practices, the respiration frequency can be reduced to 6-10 times per minute or even lower to 2-5 times. Deep and slow respiration can give

---

[12] 五脏六腑 Wu Zang Liu Fu - five internal organs/viscera (heart, lung, spleen, liver, kidney), six bowels (stomach, small and large intestines, gallbladder, bladder, and triple burner)

the respiratory organs more resting time, so they do not easily tire and minimizing gasping, heart-pounding, etc. that often appear with exertion during physical activity.

Part 2: Effects on the Digestive System

While practicing Daoist Qigong, the continuous expansion and contraction movements of the lower abdomen enhance metabolic activity within the body, resulting in a strengthening of the body's inner metabolism. As a result, the digestive organs must strengthen their functions to better absorb nutrients from food to meet the needs of the body. Therefore, after practice, the appetite increases and the taste of food is especially pleasant. During the course of breath practice, saliva (the ancients called it "divine liquid" and "spirit water") increases. At the same time as sinking the breath, swallow it into the stomach. Then, it can irrigate dirty bowels, lubricate and moisten the limbs, and also can help digestion. Practice can stimulate the digestive organs to secrete more digestive fluids, strengthen peristalsis in the stomach and intestines, and improve blood circulation. Then, food is easier to digest and absorb.

The rhythmic movement of the Dan Tian sticking out and sinking in provide a beneficial mechanical massage for the stomach, intestines, liver, and spleen. Consequently, the functions of these organs are also enhanced.

Part 3: Effects on the Nervous System

Every activity in the human body is regulated through and carried out under the nervous system. Conversely, various kinds of sports movement produce a corresponding influence in entire nervous system, improving its functions. In practicing Wudang Qigong, constant attention must be paid to the limbs of the body coordinating up and down, the inside and outside are connected as one, the heart is calm and the spirit is quiet, the mind is aware and understands subtle phenomenon. This unifies and coordinates all parts of the body with the spirit mind (shen yi). Under these conditions, the inner breath as though inside a great tunnel circulates around the large and small heavenly circles, the four limbs and hundred bones, raising, heightening, and strengthening the functions of the nervous system in control of the motor organs. Regular practice that is not lax can improve the excitation and adaptability of the nervous system, so responses to external stimulation quicken and are more precise. Resulting in greater flexibility, coordination, and integration of organ and system activities within the body. At the same time this also enhances the cerebellum's control functions, evidenced by the ability to go to sleep quickly and to sleep soundly, making it an effective treatment for neurasthenia.[13] Second, when studying, the cerebellum functions are extremely clear and alert, efficiency is high, and quality good. Regular practice of Wudang Qigong can increase the endurance and strength of the body and the functions of the cerebellum, increasing and heightening resistance to external pathogens. Then, a person need not fear rigorous cold or extreme heat, can keep away pathogens, eliminate illness, and have a long life.

Part 4: Effects on the Cardiovascular System

Practicing Daoist Qigong can help keep the cardiovascular system healthy, preventing conditions like high blood pressure, and hardening of the arteries. The distinctive movements of Daoist Qigong, characterized by spiral patterns and circular shaped movements along with the breath circulation and the Dan Tian sticking out and sinking in, all contribute to this effect.

[13] neurasthenia - an emotional and psychic disorder that is characterized by impaired functioning in interpersonal relationships and often by fatigue, depression, feelings of inadequacy, headaches, hypersensitivity to sensory stimulation (as by light or noise) and psychosomatic symptoms (as disturbances of digestion and circulation) (Webster's)

The processes of doing the movements in all directions and the extent of the movements during winding, coiling, twisting, turning with pushing down the breath, raising the breath, sinking the breath sends the breath through the internal and external movements promotes gentle dilation in the arterial blood vessels and lymph glands, thereby preserving the blood vessel and lymph gland elasticity and strengthening the unimpeded and unobstructed circulation of blood and promoting lymph functions.

Moreover, the practice leads to a relative weakening in the response of the sympathetic nerves and the response of the parasympathetic nerves is strengthened. This change in the body's reactions helps normalize vascular circulation. Consequently, refining and cultivating Daoist Qigong contributes in a positive way to slowing the results of aging on the cardiovascular system.

Section 3 Points to Pay Attention To

To learn any skill, everything must follow according to the natural principles, from shallow to deep, from simple to complex, to gradually improve. During practice, it is essential to observe the "eight requirements" and avoid the "three evils" – Do not be excessively hungry, excessively full, wantonly desire, or angry.

Part 1 Observe the 8 Requirements Avoid the 3 Mistakes

The Eight Requirements are:

1. When the heart is calm, the spirit is tranquil.
2. When the spirit is tranquil, the heart is set at ease.
3. When the heart is set at ease, it is full and still.
4. When there is fullness and stillness, there are no disturbances.
5. When there are no disturbances, the breath can circulate.
6. When the breath can circulate, one can transcend appearances.
7. When one transcends appearances, one discovers heightened awareness.
8. Heightened awareness leads the spirit and the breath to join together and ten thousand things to return to their root.

Those who do not understand the three mistakes may find it easy to fall into misguided practices, leading to disturbances in their practice. Only with understanding can the benefits be obtained. So what are these three mistakes? They are the mistakes of using brute force, overly exerting breath, lifting the chest and tucking in the abdomen. If brute force is used, the blood cannot circulate through the veins of the four limbs and hundred bones, the tendons and ligaments cannot relax, the whole body feels restricted, the hands and feet cannot be coordinated. Due to brute force, the whole body becomes stagnated and parts become sluggish and sluggishness turns into disease.

If in practice the breath is overly exerted or if the breath is too strong or energetic, it is easy to damage the lungs. Because the lungs serve to discharge stagnant breath by squeezing, it is easy to cause symptoms such as breathlessness and other lung disorders. Similarly, lifting the chest and tucking in the abdomen disrupts the natural flow of the internal breath. It cannot entirely return down to the Dan Tian and both feet seem like floating duckweed with no root. If the mind and its ruler are not in harmony, even with ten thousand methods, a person still cannot achieve harmony in the effort. So, when practicing one cannot commit "the three mistakes" of malpractice.

Part 2 Points to Pay Attention To

During practice, if one is too hungry, one will not have physical strength. If one is too full, it is easy to damage the spleen and stomach. If the thoughts are careless and random it is easy to deviate and be misled or go astray. When one is angry, the breath will be sudden and violent, not easily circulating through the large and small heavenly circles. During practice, one should not chat or laugh casually, spit saliva, or excrete urine or feces. If one chats and laughs casually, the energy and spirit disburse and it is not easy to achieve deep concentration. If one spits saliva, the mouth and the tongue become dry, water and fire cannot balance, and internal body heat increases. If one excretes urine or feces, it's easy for the breath to leak and strength to be scattered. After practice, one cannot be anxious to eat or drink, take a seat or lie down, Instead, gradually release the state. This is expressed well by the common saying: "After practice, walk one hundred steps, arrive at old age without entering a medicine shop."

In order to maintain this permanently, practice and study cannot be lax. Wudang Qigong, similar to other workmanship exercises, relies on lasting practice. Avoid the mindset of "go fishing for three days and dry the nets for two" or thinking that the exercise doctrine is too high, the exercise methods too difficult, so you feel too dull and awkward to study, or assuming the workmanship is too easy, that you already have a very high-level of mastery. Only those who practice diligently with a humble spirit, seeking guidance and striving for continuous improvement, can achieve a state of inner emptiness, a natural demeanor, and an unobstructed flow of vital energy.

Part 3 In Practice One Cannot be Obstinate

In practicing Wudang Qigong, one cannot be self-centered or obstinate. It leads to stagnation and lack of flexibility. In one who focuses solely on what is heavy, the results will be heavy not lively. In one who fixates only on the inner breath, the result will be constrained not flowing. The one who only seeks lightness, the spirit will scatter and disperse. In short, when the body's outer form is put in order, imperceptibly and naturally physical strength will increase. When the body is connected inside, imperceptibly vitality will increase.

During practice, one must also achieve respiration without a sound, inhalation and exhalation must be gradual and unbroken, resembling the subtle rhythm of "breathing and resting" neither storing nor losing, this is called true breathing. Consequently, when there is sound it is called wind breathing and even if there is no sound but the breath is not long and extended it is called thin breathing, going out and entering are sluggish this is gasping breathing. None of these align with the essence of Wudang Qigong's essential aims, because when "windedness is observed, then the breath is scattered, when thinness is observed then the breathing is hard; when gasping is observed, then the breath is congealed." So then, winded, thin, or gasping these three breaths, all cannot achieve the eight methods of: leisurely, slow, careful, well-distributed, still, continuous, deep, and long." Only if one achieves the eight methods of true breathing, then and only then will the demeanor be stable and the state of mind cheerful. If one practices until the exercise is perfected, when concentrating on the lower Dan Tian, the body will naturally become as heavy as Mount Tai and the energy and the inner breath will combine, changing to become completely empty, so the body will naturally feel light as a feather. Thus when practicing do not stubbornly cling to one aspect. If one understands the mystery, it seems to become a state of both presence and absence, without attachments, both real and unreal. This understanding comes effortlessly, without conscious thought, and seamlessly enters the Tao without form yet alive. Earlier teachers said: “Energy gives birth to agility, root breath gives birth to the spirit, the path of Daoist Qigong is true. Dan tian practice creates a long-life treasure that ten thousand measures of yellow gold cannot give a person."

Wudang Daoist Qigong's profound principles are high

Diligently study, practice from memory, careful and deliberate

With unceasing workmanship, study each method oneself,

After a considerable period of time, then see rare effects.

Section 4 Wudang Qigong 18 Exercises to Refine the Breath

Inner breath circulation, acupuncture points, and discharging from the bone all have refining the inner breath and cultivating the body at their foundation. According to what has been handed down by many teachers, collect and gather earlier Heaven's inner breath, practice the forms and methods moving, sitting, lying down, apply the method of abiding without clinging, then the inner breath follows the large heavenly circle the small heavenly circle and the tiny heavenly circle, to refine the character and cultivate true vision, progressing from the realm of delusion and intention action to non-action.

The twelve meridians and eight extraordinary vessels in the human body are closely connected to the five viscera and six bowels. The Yin channel flows through the internal organs and the Yang channel flows through the viscera. Qigong masters and martial arts experts can treat illness and cure disease, use pressure points to check the inner breath, adjust damage to viscera and internal organs, all because they understand the various points along the meridians and channels.

When beginning to practice China's Wudang Daoist Breath Exercises, on breathing in push the tongue against the upper palate; on breathing out the tongue rests on the lower palate. Once the circulation of inner breath and blood is unobstructed and smooth, the position of the tongue against the upper palate does not change.

Set 1 Extreme Emptiness Exercise

Extreme emptiness method combines heaven and earth,
Completely empty without appearances
raise the crown of the head
The intention is at the Lao Gong raise the Yong Quan,
empty the mind, fill the belly and the breath will rise.

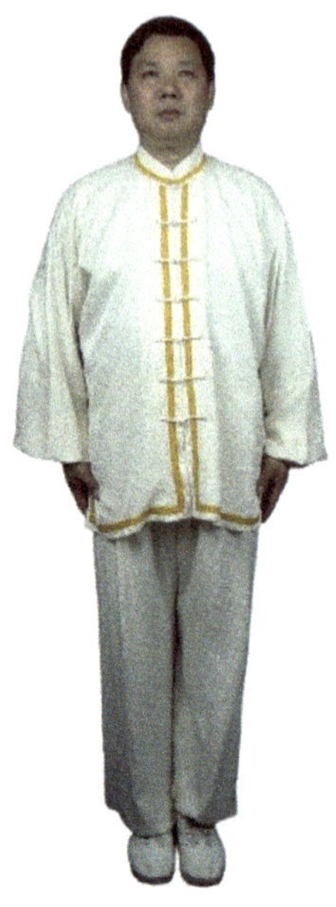

Illustration 1-1 Preparation Posture

1) Preparation

The body faces south standing straight with the two feet together, both arms naturally hang down, the index finger is slightly raised. The eyes look front, the intention is on the palm, Lao Gong acupuncture point. (Illustration 1-1)

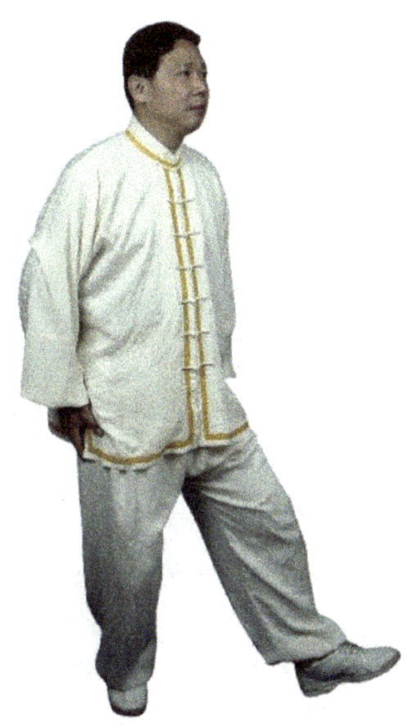

Illustration 1-2 Preparation Posture

After naturally breathing out and breathing in two times, the body turns left 45 degrees. The heel of the left foot presses along the ground toward the left side pushing out 30 centimeters, the toes close inward, the toes grip the ground, the center of the foot, the Yong Quan acupuncture point, raises upward. The eyes follow the body's movement, the intention is on the Yong Quan, the breath circulates through the foot's Jue Yin Gan channel. (Illustration 1-2)

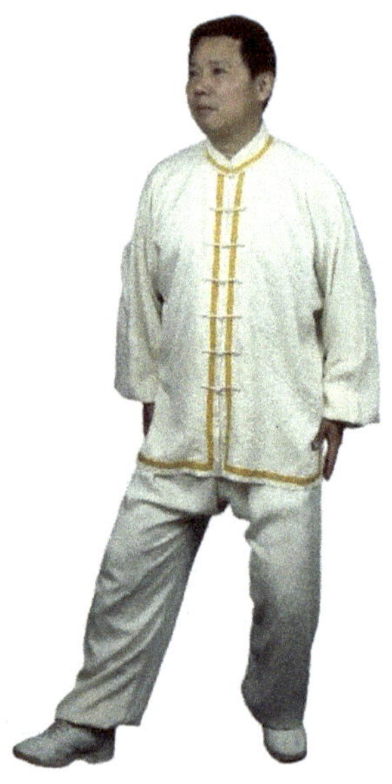

Illustration 1-3 Preparation Posture

The previous movement pauses slightly, the center of gravity shifts left, the body turns toward the right 90 degrees, the heel of the right foot presses along the ground toward the right pushing out 15 centimeters, the right toes close to the inside and press on the ground. The eyes follow the turning of the body, the intention is on the Xuan Guan opening. (Illustration 1-3)

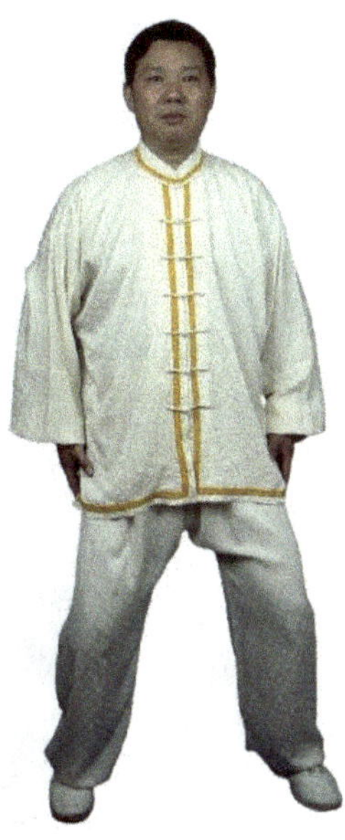

Illustration 1-4 Preparation Posture

The previous movement does not stop, the body turns toward the left 45 degrees, still facing South and standing straight, the lower jaw is slightly drawn back, at the crown of the head the Bai Hui acupuncture point raises upward; empty the mind, fill the belly, and breathe naturally. The eyes look forward, the intention observes the lower Dan Tian. (Illustration 1-4)

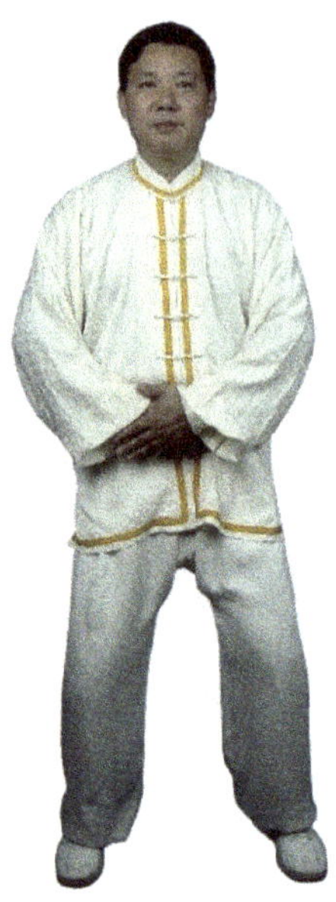

Illustration 1-5 Raise Upward and Rub Downward

2) Raise Upward and Rub Downward

After circulating the breath two times, both hands from the sides of the body follow an arc in front of the abdomen. The palms face inward, (because yin and yang in men and women are not the same) women have the right hand outside, men have the left hand outside, the Lao Gong of both hands fold together and press against each other, lightly pressing above the lower Dan Tian (the place 4.2 centimeters below the naval also known as the Qi Hai acupuncture point). The eyes look slightly downward, the intention observes the Dan Tian. (Illustration 1-5)

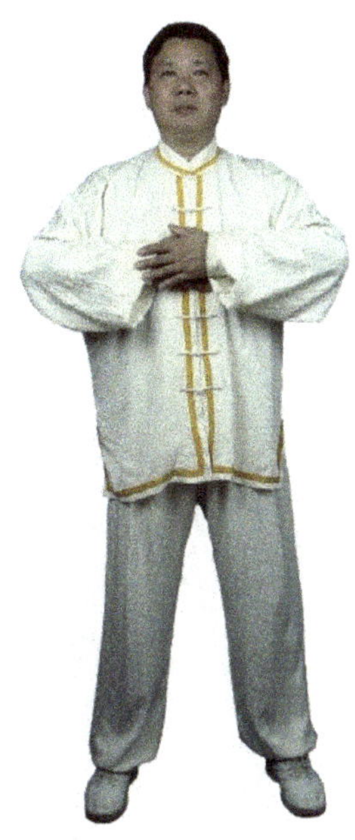

Illustration 1-6 Raise Upward and Rub Downward

The previous movement does not stop, both arms slightly revolve outward, the palms face inward and stick to the body traveling upward and stopping in front of the chest. The center of the palms Lao Gong acupuncture points and the center between the two breasts, the Tanzhong acupuncture point, are aligned and attract each other. At the same time, the Dan Tian sinks inward, breathe in. The tongue presses against the upper palate, the teeth are slightly closed, the eyes look front, the intention observes the Lao Gong acupuncture points. (Illustration 1-6)

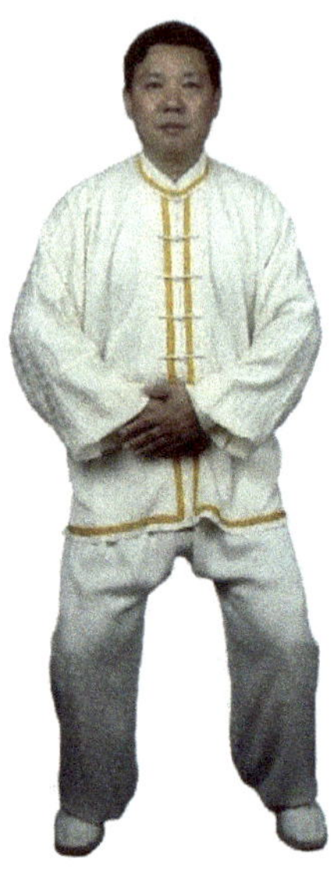

Illustration 1-7 Raise Upward and Rub Downward

The previous movement pauses, the body's center of gravity lowers, both legs bend at the knees and squat down changing to a horse stance. At the same time, both arms slightly revolve inward, the palms face downward at an angle, sticking to the body and smoothly moving downward, stopping in front of the navel. At the same time, the Dan Tian sticks outward, breathe out (practice until the breath sinks to the Dan Tian, then when breathing out and breathing in the tongue presses against the upper palate, don't use the repeated up and down movement). The tongue rests on the lower palate, the teeth are lightly closed. The eyes look front, the intention observes the Bai Hui. (Illustration 1-7)

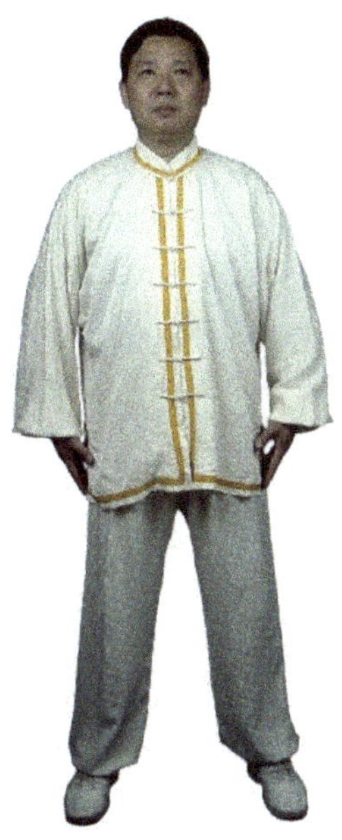

Illustration 1-8 Blend the Elements with One Breath

3) Blend the Elements with One Breath

The previous movement pauses slightly. After circulating the breath out and in two times, both legs extend to stand naturally. At the same time, both hands from the front of the body open and turn downwards in an arc stopping at the sides of the body. The eyes look forward and the intention is at the Dan Tian. (Illustration 1-8)

Main Points and Functions

Extreme Emptiness Exercise main point is to refine and cultivate the Dan Tian inner breath. When breathing in, the center of the foot Yong Quan acupuncture point, the centers of the palms Lao Gong acupuncture points, the center at the crown of the head Bai Hui acupuncture point, these three centers breathe in from above, the middle, and below (yang, middle, yin) returning the three inner breaths to the Dan Tian. The middles of the three centers have a slightly cool, numb, or tingling feeling. When breathing out from the three centers to discharge the breath, the three centers have a slightly warm feeling (after practicing this skill for 100 days, the warm feeling will increase). When the Breath in the Dan Tian is sufficient, as a matter of course, the energy and inner breath will circulate through the large and small heavenly circles. For beginners just learning Wudang Daoist Qigong, if the breath does not seem very deep, concentrate the intention on observing the center of the Lao Gong acupuncture points, paying attention to regulating the breathing. When breathing in and raising the arms, the shoulders must relax, the elbows must sink down. When pressing down and breathing out, the feet must sustain and the hips must sit. The sphincter near the Hui Yin must lift up. In revealing the secret it is said: "Tightly bring together the anus lifting from inside, with clear eyes brilliant rise flying to the top." The intention observes the breath in the Dan Tian with the thoughts not accepting any outside interference. When the spirit and form join together and harmonize a person can live longer. Extreme Emptiness is the beginning of a practice to build inner strength that can enable one who practices to gradually achieve a practice in which the spirit returns to emptiness, returning to nothing (无极 Wu Ji) the most advanced and highest state.

Practice Method

Each time, practice 6 times or 9 times to make one set, practicing again and again in succession is fine. The extent of the movement being larger or smaller, moving higher or lower is without restriction, depending on the age of the person practicing being older or younger, whether the physical force is greater or lesser, and the weakness or strength in the body.

Acupuncture Points 点穴 (dian xue)

Lao Gong xue 劳宫穴 Palace of Toil PC-8[who]

Yong Quan xue 涌泉穴 Bubbling Spring KC-1[who]

Tan Zhong xue 膻中穴 Chest Center CV-17[who]

Jue Yin Gan jing 厥阴肝经 Reverting Yin Liver channel

Xuan Guan qiao 玄关窍 Mysterious Gate (upper Dan Tian)

Bai Hui xue 百会穴 Hundred Convergences GV-20[who]

Qi Hai 气海 Sea of Qi CV-6[who]

Set 2 Pushing the Mountain Exercise

In Pushing the Mountain

the inner breath gathers in the Dan Tian,

Issuing or receiving, circulating and transforming

do not change the countenance.

The triple burner is unimpeded, the breath is not obstructed,

strengthen the body, guard the health,

protect the original breath.[14]

[14] 真元 zhen yuan - true breath; 元气 yuan qi - original breath

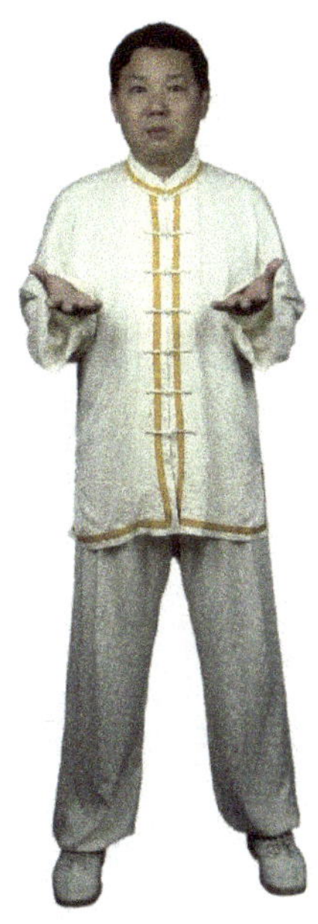

Illustration 2-1 Extremely Empty Initially

1) Preparation

These movement methods are exactly the same as for Extreme Emptiness Exercise, Preparation Postures. (see Illustrations 1-1, 1-2, 1-3, 1-4)

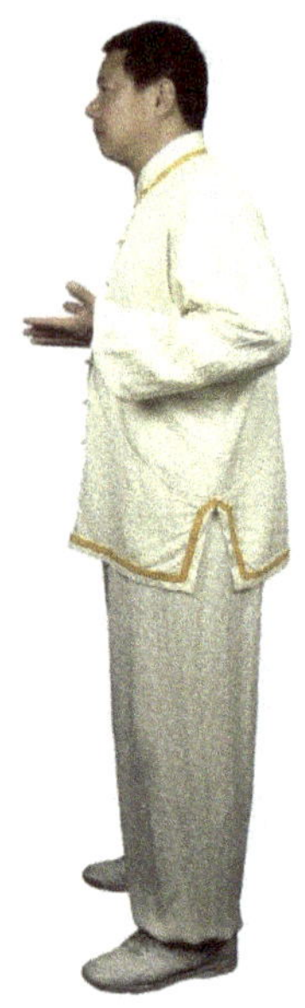

Illustration 2-2 Extremely Empty Initially

2) Extremely Empty Initially

The previous movement pauses slightly. After circulating the breath out and in two times, both legs extend to stand naturally. At the same time, both arms revolve to the outside; both hands together turn inward and rise upward, the heels of the palms stop just below both breasts. The fingertips of both hands point front, the palms face up. At the same time, the Dan Tian sinks inward, breathe in. The tongue rises against the upper palate, the teeth are slightly closed, the eyes look to the front. (Illustrations 2-1 and 2-2)

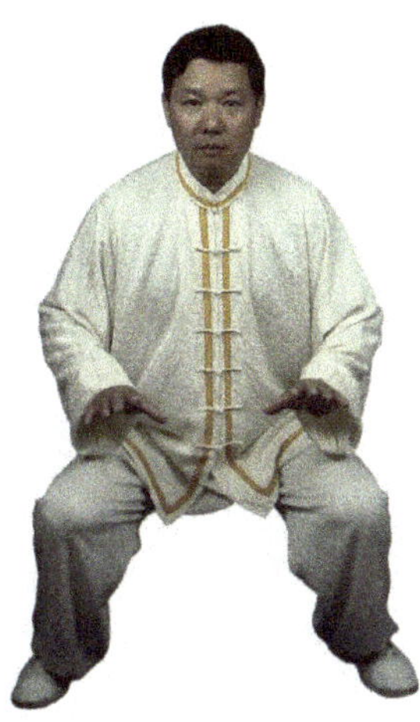

Illustration 2-3 Extremely Empty Initially

The previous movement does not stop, the body's center of gravity lowers, both legs bend at the knees to squat down changing to a horse stance. At the same time, both arms revolve inward and both elbows hold together, the hands turn toward the front of the body in an arc shape and press down, stopping in front of the abdomen. The palms face down, the fingertips point forward. At the same time, the Dan Tian sticks outward, breathe out. The tongue rests on the lower palate; the teeth are lightly closed. The eyes look slightly downward; the intention is at the Dan Tian, the breath circulates through both the Du Mai and the Ren Mai. (Illustration 2-3)

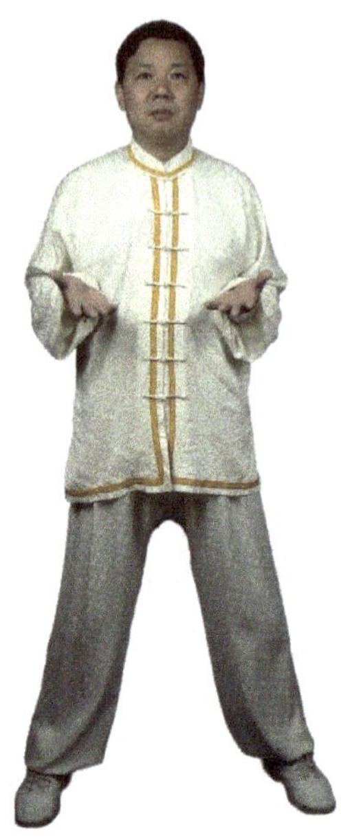

Illustration 2-4 Pushing the Mountain Exercise

3) Pushing the Mountain Exercise

The previous movement pauses slightly. After circulating the breath out and in two times, both legs extend to stand naturally. At the same time, both arms revolve to the outside; both hands together turn inward and rise upward, the heels of the palms stop just below both breasts. The fingertips of both hands point front, the palms face up. At the same time, the Dan Tian sinks inward, breathe in. The tongue rises against the upper palate, the teeth are slightly closed, the eyes look to the front. (Illustration2-4)

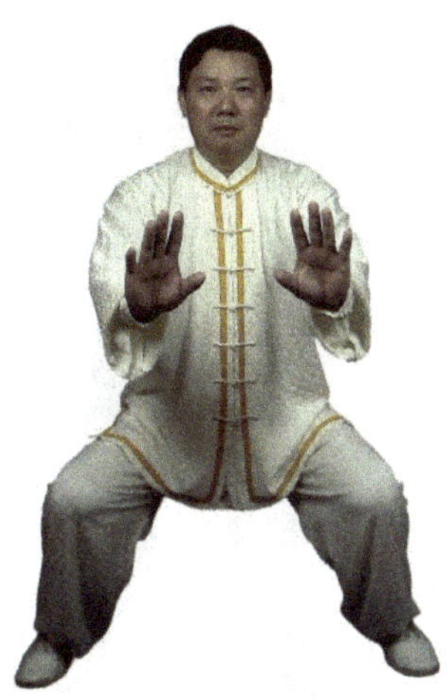

Illustration 2-5 Pushing the Mountain Exercise

The previous movement does not stop, the body's center of gravity lowers, both legs bend at the knees to squat down, changing into a horse stance. At the same time, both arms revolve inward, the heels of the palms use strength, pushing toward the front along a level plane. The distance between the centers of the two palms and the centers of both breasts is the same width, the palms face forward the fingertips point up. Also at the same time, the Dan Tian sticks out, gradually breathe out. The tongue rests on the lower palate, the teeth are lightly closed. The eyes look through the center of the space between both palms toward the front and into the distance, the intention is on the palms Lao Gong acupuncture points. (Illustration 2-5)

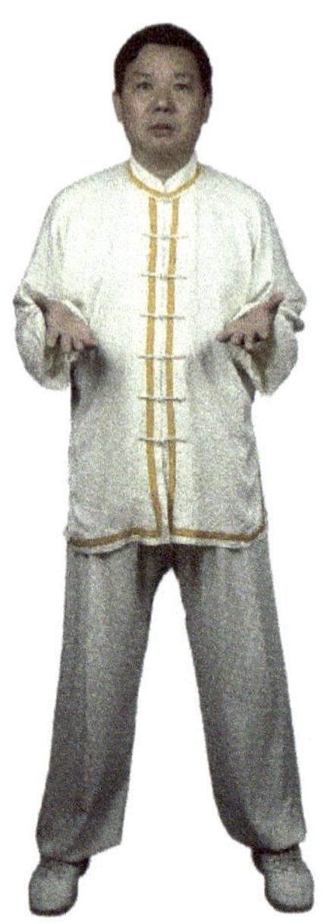

Illustration 2-6 Blend the Elements with One Breath

4) Blend the Elements with One Breath

The previous movement pauses slightly. After circulating the breath out and in two times, both legs extend to stand naturally. At the same time, both arms revolve to the outside; both hands together turn inward and rise upward, the heels of the palms stop just below both breasts. The fingertips of both hands point front, the palms face up. At the same time, the Dan Tian sinks inward, breathe in. The tongue rises against the upper palate, the teeth are slightly closed, the eyes look to the front. (Illustration 2-6)

These movements are entirely the same as Extreme Emptiness Exercise, Blend the Elements with One Breath (see Illustration 1-8).

Main Points and Functions

The important point in practicing Pushing the Mountain Exercise is that the Lao Gong acupuncture points turn outward and send out inner breath. In the very beginning the shapeless and formless "Dao" created and sent out true original breath. True breath separates yin and yang, yin and yang develop and produce the three cai, four directions, five elements, eight trigrams thereby giving birth to and transforming ten thousand things. Thus, returning to the original source and achieving the objective of a healthy body and long life. When raising the arms and breathing out, the shoulders must relax and the elbows must sink. The movement and the breathing must be closely coordinated, fully complete, when the hands stop, the breath in must be full. Hold the spirit inside, relax the whole body, Observe the energy and spirit inside, relax the whole body, the toes grip the ground, and the inner breath travels upward. The upper body is straight, the Hui Yin acupuncture point and the crown of the head center the Bai Hui acupuncture point shine from above and below.

When breathing out, it should be synchronized with the lowering of the body, the speed slow and even. When the Lao Gong acupuncture points face out, send out the inner breath and push with the palms, the appearance is the same as if pushing a piece of wood on the water; or very much like the appearance of pushing a ball in the water. The whole body is shrouded in a type of "outer breath" and covered by it, with unregulated inner breath. Use the intention to send out the inner breath, neither excessively extending nor not reaching. Use the method of neither expecting nor overly exerting, then it is possible to send out the inner breath and perform the exercise.

Practice Method

Each time, practice 6 times or 9 times to make one set, practicing again and again in succession is fine. The extent of the movement being larger or smaller, moving higher or lower is without restriction, depending on the age of the person practicing being older or younger, whether the physical strength is greater or lesser, and the weakness or strength in the body.

Acupuncture Points 点穴 (dian xue)

Zhen Yuan 真元 True Breath.

Yuan Qi 元气 Original Breath

Du Mai 督脉 Governing Vessel GV[who]

Ren Mai 任脉 Controlling Vessel; Conception Vessel CV[who]

Hui Yin 会阴 Meeting of Yin (perineum) CV-1[who]

Set 3 Wild Goose Flying Exercise

Wild geese spread their wings to soar into the open sky,
a wild swan lowers to the earth, refining the inner Dan
The breath passes through both arms, raise both heels,
fly upward and lower downward quietly, noiselessly.

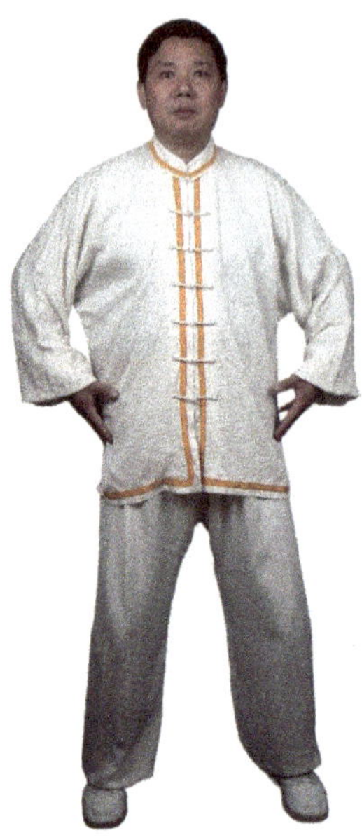

Illustration 3-1 Nestling Swallow Learns to Fly

1) Preparation

These movement methods are exactly the same as for Extreme Emptiness Exercise, Preparation Postures. (see Illustrations 1-1, 1-2, 1-3, 1-4)

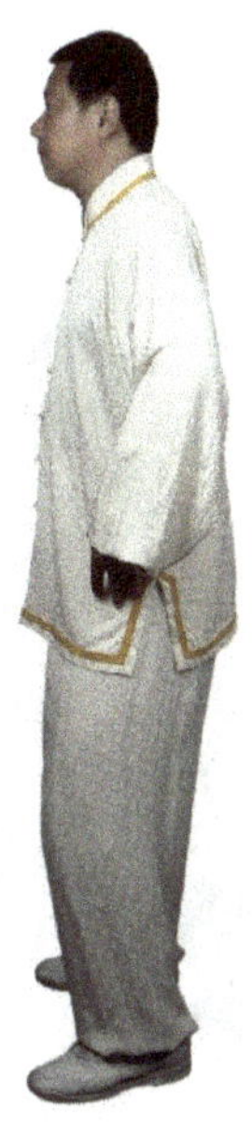

Illustration 3-2 Nestling Swallow Learns to Fly

2) Nestling Swallow Learns to Fly

The previous movement does not stop, both hands from the sides of the body move upward in an arc, stopping at the waist, the fingertips of the hands point at the Zhang Men acupuncture points, the palms Lao Gong acupuncture points withdraw inward, both elbows open to the outside, both arms bend like a new moon. The shoulders relax, the elbows sink down. Also at the same time, the Dan Tian sinks inward, breathe in. The tip of the tongue presses against the upper palate, the teeth are slightly closed. The eyes look inside, the intention observes the center between both eyes, the Xuan Guan opening. (Illustrations 3-1, 3-2)

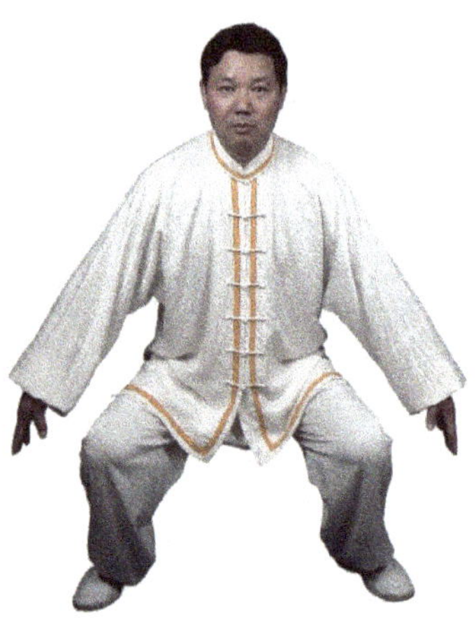

Illustration 3-3 Nestling Swallow Learns to Fly

The previous movement pauses slightly, the body's center of gravity lowers, both legs bend at the knees to squat down changing to a horse stance. At the same time, both arms revolve inward, both hands brush the spleen and liver descending along both sides of the legs. The palms face each other, the fingertips point diagonally to the ground (if when one is practicing, the lower back is not comfortable, both hands should massage the kidneys when descending). Also at the same time, the Dan Tian sticks outward, breathe out. The tongue rests on the lower palate, the teeth are lightly closed. The eyes look downward slightly, the intention is on connecting yin and yang, upper and lower. (Illustration 3-3)

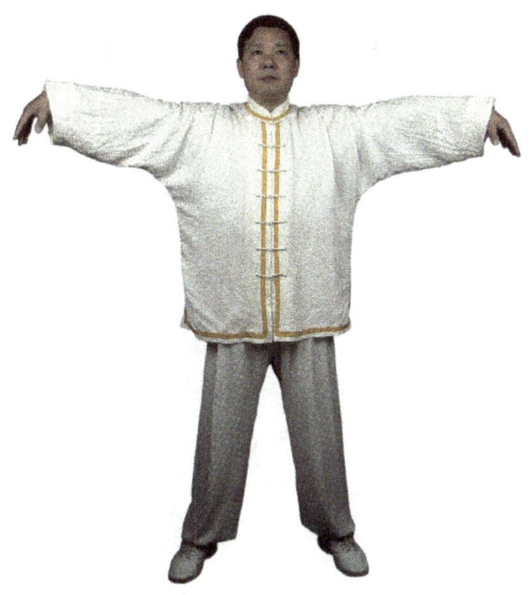

Illustration 3-4 Up and Down Spread the Wings

3) Up and Down Spread the Wings

The previous movement pauses slightly, the heels raise up, both legs stretch straight, the body rises straight up. At the same time, both hands from the front of the body turn toward the sides of the body, rising upward in an arc shape, the fingertips point downward at an angle, both wrist joints rise upward using strength, slightly higher than the shoulders. Also at the same time, the Dan Tian sinks inward, breathe in. The chest is open and the breath smooth, the tip of the tongue presses against the upper palate, the teeth are slightly closed. The eyes look toward the front and up, the intention is on the Dan Tian breath rising along the Du Mai and traveling up to the center at the crown of the head, the Bai Hui acupuncture point. The whole body has a feeling of flying into the blue sky and going directly to the Golden Top Palace. (Illustration 3-4)

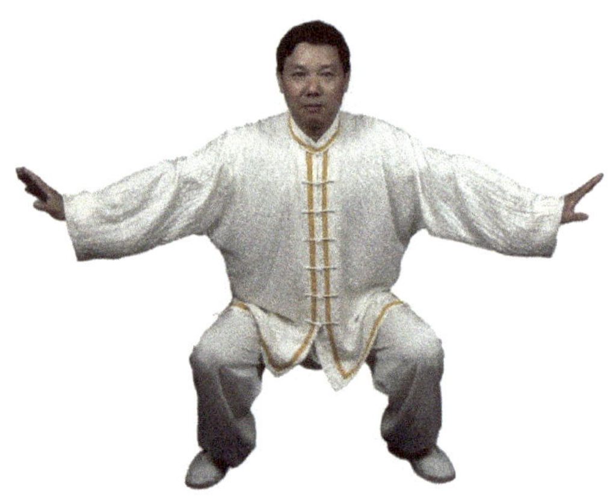

Illustration 3-5 Up and Down Spread the Wings

The previous movement does not stop, the body's center of gravity sinks down, the heels remain on the ground, both legs bend at the knees to squat down, changing to a horse stance. At the same time, the wrists sit down, both arms gradually lower, stopping at the sides of the body. The fingertips point out; the palms face down at an angle. At the same time, the Dan Tian sticks outward, breathe out. The tongue rests on the lower palate, the teeth are lightly closed. The eyes look toward the front, the intention is on sinking down the bend of the elbows Qu Chi acupuncture point. The whole body is permeated with inner breath, appearing the same as a flock of wild geese settling onto a sandy beach, comfortable without comparison. (Illustration 3-5)

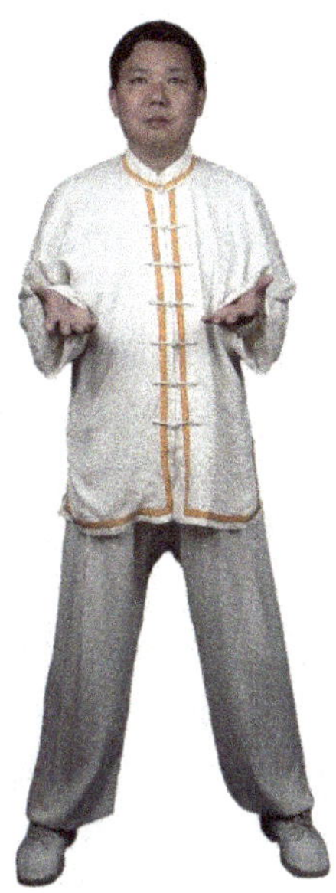

Illustration 3-6 Blend the Elements with One Breath

4) Blend the Elements with One Breath

The previous movement pauses slightly. After circulating the breath out and in two times, both legs extend to stand naturally. At the same time, both arms revolve to the outside; both hands together turn inward and rise upward, the heels of the palms stop just below both breasts. The fingertips of both hands point front, the palms face up. At the same time, the Dan Tian sinks inward, breathe in. The tongue rises against the upper palate, the teeth are slightly closed, the eyes look to the front. (Illustration 3-6)

These movements are entirely the same as Extreme Emptiness Exercise, Blend the Elements with One Breath (see Illustration 1-8).

Main Points and Functions

Swallow Flying Exercise, because it combines rising and settling, circulating the breath is the core, it is one way of using breathing mainly as a method to develop internal workmanship. When raising the arms upward to fly, pay attention to the head rising straight upward, the soles of the feet pressing on the earth, the body extending unanimously while simultaneously using the whole body, having the same appearance as though flying up into the sky. The centers of the feet Yong Quan acupuncture points with the Bai Hui acupuncture point reflect each other. breathing in must be gradual, slow, careful, and long like pulling out a silk thread, namely long, well-distributed and not broken. When lowering downward, the toes of the feet grab the earth, the Yong Quan acupuncture points raise upward, the body above and below is linked as one, the joints are open, press down slowly and evenly. When the shoulders are relaxed, the inner breath sinks to the elbows, when the elbow sinks, the inner breath travels down to the wrist, when the writ sits the inner breath passes through the fingertips. When the hips relax, the inner breath travels down to the knees, when the knees are bent, the inner breath travels down to the Yong Quan.

When circulating the inner breath, requires concentrated attention and complete consideration, to achieve: soft, slow, uniform, long, and deep. Soft, breathing is light and fine. Slow, taking in breath and breathing out are gradual and slow. Uniform, the rhythm of the breath is even. Long, the breath interval is longer. Deep, the breath penetrates through the four limbs and hundred bones, circulating through the whole body.

Practice Method

Each time, practice 6 times or 9 times to make one set, practicing again and again in succession is fine. The extent of the movement being larger or smaller, moving higher or lower is without restriction, depending on the age of the person practicing being older or younger, whether the physical strength is greater or lesser, and the weakness or strength in the body.

Acupuncture Points 点穴 (dian xue)

Zhang Men xue 章门穴 Camphorwood Gate LV-13

Lao Gong xue 劳宫穴 Palace of Toil PC-8[who]

Xuan Guan qiao 玄关窍 Mysterious Gate (upper Dan Tian)

Du Mai 督脉 Governing Vessel GV[who]

Bai Hui xue 百会穴 Hundred Convergences GV-20[who]

Qu Chi xue 曲池穴 Pool at the Bend LI-11[who]

Yong Quan xue 涌泉穴 Bubbling Spring KC-1[who]

Set 4 Bending Crane Exercise

The person who practices White Crane Skill has long life,
diagonally soaring, the body moves like a gentle breeze.
View the myriad things of the world as dust,
organically the spirit and breath join.

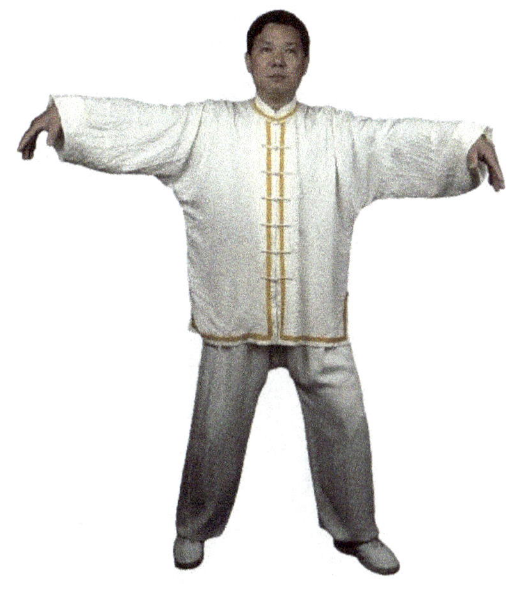

Illustration 4-1 Left Bend and Fly

1) Preparation

These movement methods are exactly the same as for Extreme Emptiness Exercise, Preparation Postures. (see Illustrations 1-1, 1-2, 1-3, 1-4)

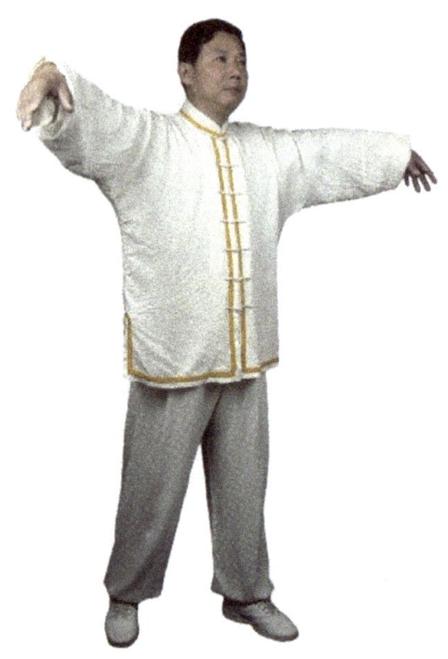

Illustration 4-2 Left Bend and Fly

2) Left Bend and Fly

The previous movement pauses slightly, after regulating the breath by breathing out and in two times, the body turns to the left 45 degrees, the weight is left six right four, the right foot heel raises changing to a left six four stance. At the same time, the body rises up to the left and unfolds, both arms follow the changes in the body's movement, gradually rising from the sides of the body to the left in an arc and slowly flying, the shoulders relax, the elbows sink down; the wrists press up with strength, slightly higher than the shoulders. The fingertips point downward at an angle to the ground, the palms face inward, the Lao Gong acupuncture points are connected from a distance with the foot San Li acupuncture points. At the same time, the Dan Tian sinks inward, breathe in. The tip of the tongue presses against the upper palate; the teeth are slightly closed. The eyes follow the body movement, the intention is at the left wrist Nei Guan and Wai Guan acupuncture points. (Illustrations 4-1 and 4-2)

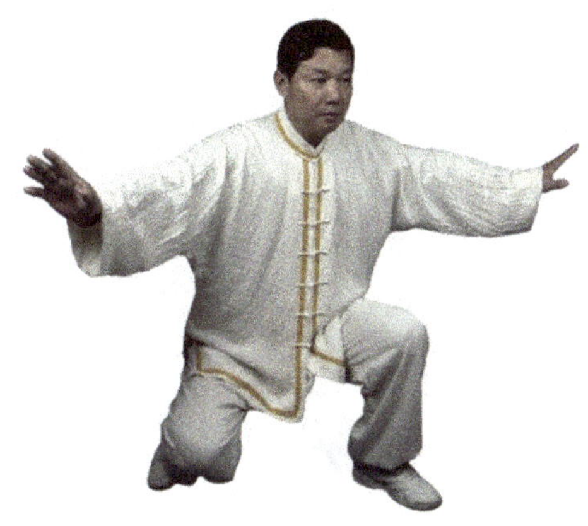

Illustration 4-3 Left Bend and Fly

The previous movement does not stop, the body's center of gravity lowers, both legs bend at the knees to squat down changing to a left six four stance. At the same time, both wrist joints bend down, both arms lower stopping at both sides of the body. The fingertips point up at an angle, the palms face down. Also at the same time, the Dan Tian sticks outward, breathe out. The tongue rests on the lower palate, the teeth are lightly closed. The eyes look into the distance, the intention is on the tip of the middle finger Zhong Chong acupuncture point, the inner breath travels through the hand Jue Yin Xin Bao channel. (Illustration 4-3)

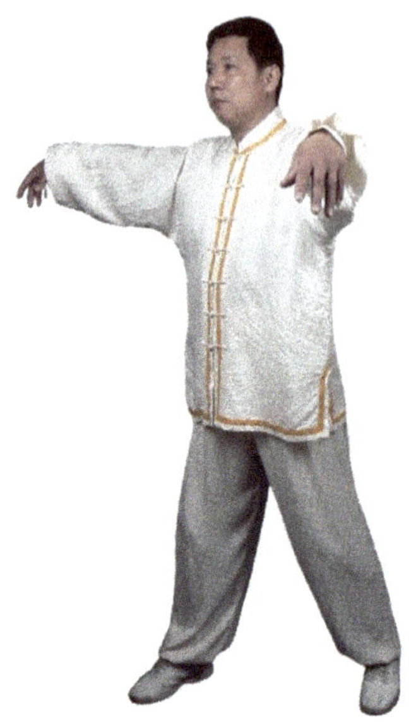

Illustration 4-4 Right Bend and Fly

3) Right Bend and Fly

The previous movement pauses slightly, the body turns right 90 degrees, the weight is right six left four, the left foot heel rises and lifts changing to a right six four stance. At the same time, the body turns toward the right and rises describing an arc, the shoulders relax, the elbows sink down, the wrist joints use strength to rise up, slightly higher than the shoulders. The fingertips point at the ground at an angle, the palms face inward, the Lao Gong acupuncture points are connected from a distance with the foot San Li acupuncture points attracting and pressing against each other. At the same time, the Dan Tian sinks inward, breathe in. The tip of the tongue presses against the upper palate; the teeth are slightly closed. The eyes follow the body movement, the intention is on the right wrist Nei Guan and Wai Guan acupuncture points. (Illustration 4-4)

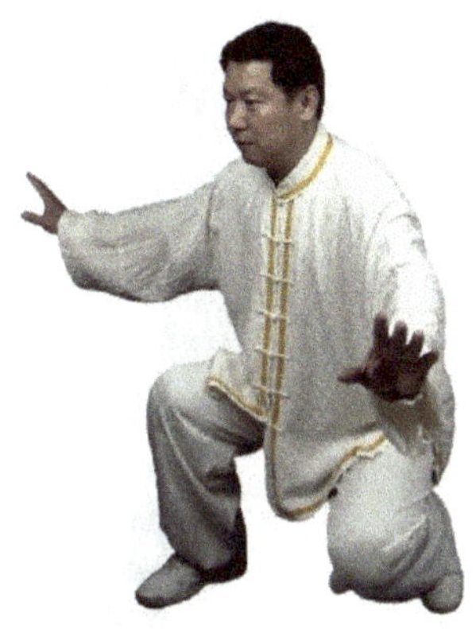

Illustration 4-5 Right Bend and Fly

The previous movement does not stop, the body's center of gravity lowers, both legs bend at the knees to squat down changing to a right six four stance. At the same time, both wrist joints sink down, both arms lower down at an angle stopping at both sides of the body. The palms face down, the fingertips angle upward. At the same time, the Dan Tian sticks outward, breathe out. The tongue rests on the lower palate, the teeth are lightly closed. The eyes look toward the front, the intention is at the tip of the middle finger Zhong Chong acupuncture point, the inner breath travels through the hand Jue Yin Xin Bao channel (Illustration 4-5)

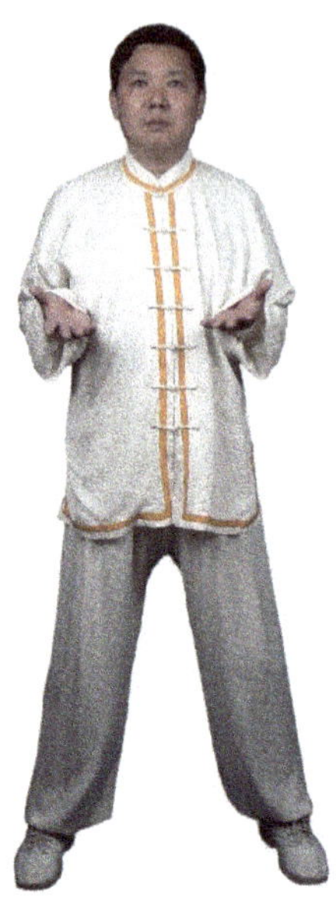

Illustration 4-6 Turn the Body Return to Beginning

4) Turn the Body Return to the Beginning

The previous movement pauses slightly. After circulating the breath out and in two times, both legs extend to stand naturally. At the same time, both arms revolve to the outside; both hands together turn inward and rise upward, the heels of the palms stop just below both breasts. The fingertips of both hands point front, the palms face up. At the same time, the Dan Tian sinks inward, breathe in. The tongue rises against the upper palate, the teeth are slightly closed, the eyes look to the front. (Illustration 4-6)

These movements are entirely the same as Extreme Emptiness Exercise, Blend the Elements with One Breath (see Illustration 1-8).

Main Points and Functions

In practicing Crane Bending Skill, all of the movements must be connected and coordinated, when the body turns the waist must be the axle, the body must be held and supported correctly, not forward, down, back or up, leaning to the left or right. The backs of the hands bend naturally, the rise and fall of the wrists must follow the movement rising and use strength to raise up, with the descending movement while sitting the wrist and raising the fingers. Inhale through the whole movement of turning the body and rising, exhale when the body center is lowering and sinking, it must be even and natural, it cannot be forced.

When practicing, also pay attention to the three straight alignments: when the neck is naturally straight, then the inner breath can permeate and infuse the Bai Hui acupuncture point; when the waist is straight and the body is relaxed, the inner breath can permeate and infuse the four limbs; when the knees are bent, the inner breath is tranquil and the spirit preserved.

Crane Diagonal Exercise is a primary workmanship method for practicing energy, qi and spirit. The length of a person's lifetime is all connected to the fullness or deficiency of energy, inner breath, and spirit. Resolutely and frequently, maintain a lasting practice, then the energy will be full, the breath complete and the spirit vigorous.

Practice Method:

Each time, practice 6 times or 12 times to make one set, practicing again and again in succession is fine. The extent of the movement being larger or smaller, moving higher or lower is without restriction, depending on the age of the person practicing being older or younger, whether the physical strength is greater or lesser, and the weakness or strength in the body.

Acupuncture Points 点穴 (dian xue)

Lao Gong xue 劳宫穴 Palace of Toil PC-8[who]

San Li xue 三里 Three Li ST-36

Nei Guan 内关 Inner Pass PC-6[who]

Wai Guan 外关 Outer Pass TB-5

Zhong Chong 中冲 Central Hub PC-9[who]

Jue Yin Xin Bao jing 厥阴心包经 Reverting Yin Pericardium channel PC[who]

Bai Hui xue 百会穴 Hundred Convergences GV-20[who]

Set 5 Supporting Heaven Exercise

Supporting Heaven raises the cauldron[15]

in the spine and extremities,

from within what seems a trance, the thoughts focus.

Xuan Zu[16] *sits steadily at the Golden Top Palace,*

nothingness inside strengthens the golden pill.[17]

---

[15] 鼎 ding - ancient cooking vessel; tripod

[16] 玄祖 Xuan Zu – Mysterious ancestor; another name for Lao Zi

[17] 丹 dan (dan tian) Cinnabar Field

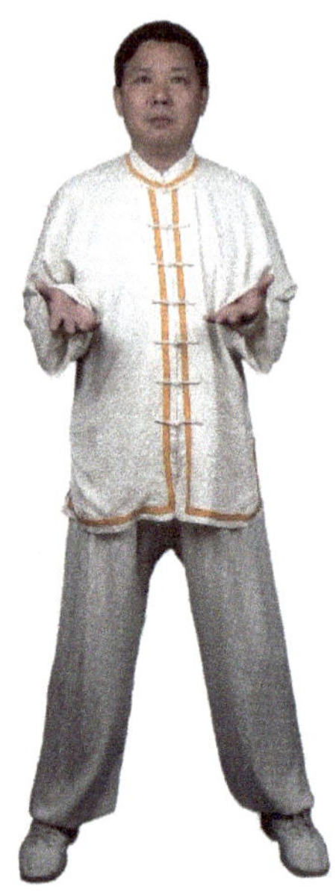

Illustration 5-1 Yin Presses Down, Yang Pushes Up

1) Preparation

These movement methods are exactly the same as for Extreme Emptiness Exercise, Preparation Postures. (see Illustrations 1-1, 1-2, 1-3, 1-4)

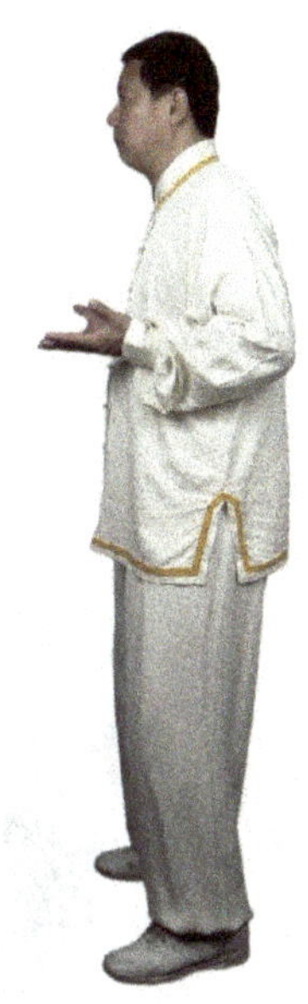

Illustration 5-2 Yin Presses Down, Yang Pushes Up

2) Yin Presses Down, Yang Pushes Up

The previous movement pauses slightly. After circulating the breath out and in two times, both legs extend to stand naturally. At the same time, both arms revolve to the outside; both hands together turn inward and rise upward, the heels of the palms stop just below both breasts. The fingertips of both hands point front, the palms face up. At the same time, the Dan Tian sinks inward, breathe in. The tongue rises against the upper palate, the teeth are slightly closed, the eyes look to the front. (Illustrations 5-1 and 5-2)

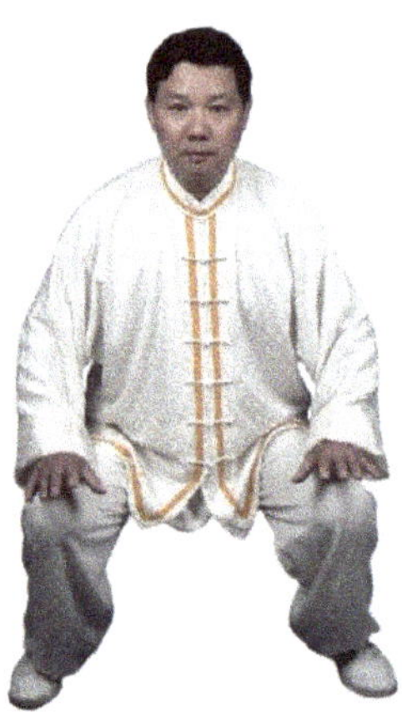

Illustration 5-3 Yin Presses Down, Yang Pushes Up

The previous movement does not stop, the body's center of gravity lowers, both legs bend at the knees to squat down changing to a horse stance. At the same time, both arms revolve inward and both elbows hold together, the hands turn toward the front of the body in an arc shape and press down, stopping in front of the abdomen. The palms face down, the fingertips point forward. At the same time, the Dan Tian sticks outward, breathe out. The tongue rests on the lower palate; the teeth are lightly closed. The eyes look slightly downward; the intention is at the Dan Tian, the breath circulates through both the Du Mai and the Ren Mai. (Illustration 5-3)

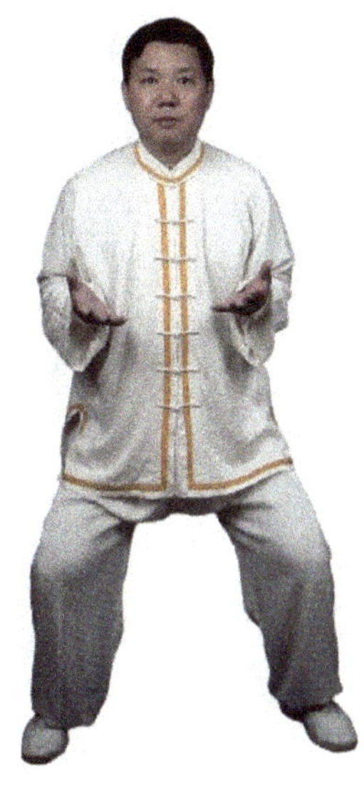

Illustration 5-4 Support Heaven, Strengthen the Dan

3) Support Heaven, Strengthen the Dan

The previous movement pauses slightly, both legs extend, the body standing naturally straight. Both arms revolve outward and turn upward, both hands follow turning upward in an arc, the heels of the palms align above the front of the chest Shen Feng acupuncture point. The palms face upward, the fingertips point forward and upward at an angle. (Illustration 5-4)

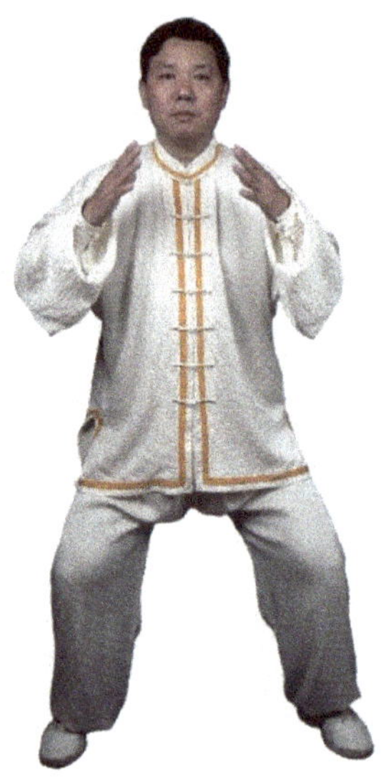

Illustration 5-5 Support the Sky, Strengthen the Dan

Just after the previous movement, both legs bend slightly to squat down, changing to a high horse stance. Both elbows support and connect with each other, the fingertips turn outward and up, both palms draw closer together, the palms face each other. The first part and the second part of this movement are both done with one breath in, it's all done in one breath. The Dan Tian sinks inward, gradually breathe in. The tongue presses against the upper palate, the teeth are slightly closed. The eyes look at the Lao Gong acupuncture points, the intention is on the Xuan Guan opening. (Illustration 5-5)

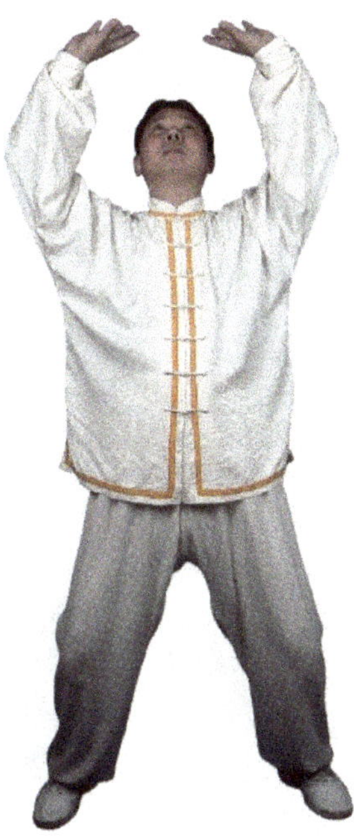

Illustration 5-6 Support the Sky, Strengthen the Dan

The previous movement does not stop, both legs extend straight, the body rises vertically. Both arms revolve inward and turn upward, both hands push up and change into yang palms, the palms face up, the fingertips point towards each other and push upward to support the sky, stopping above the top of the head. Also at the same time, the Dan Tian sticks outward, breathe out. The tongue rests on the lower palate, the teeth are lightly closed. The body slightly inclines back, the eyes from the centers of both eyes look upward into the distance, the intention is on the front of the head Shen Ting acupuncture point. (Illustration 5-6)

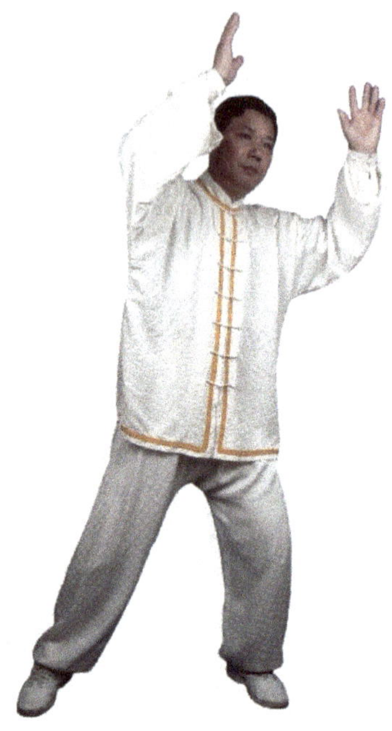

Illustration 5-7 Heavenly Dragon Waves its Tail

4) Heavenly Dragon Waves its Tail

The previous movement pauses slightly, both arms revolve outward, both hands lower in a smooth motion, the fingertips are up, the palm Lao Gong acupuncture points face each other. Both hands are 30 centimeters apart, they stop in front of the left side of the forehead. At the same time, using the waist as an axle, sway the body to the left and slightly sinking the body's center of gravity into a left six right four stance. (Illustration 5-7)

The previous movement does not stop, using the waist as an axle, sway the whole body to the right, the body's center of gravity continues to lower into a right six right four stance.

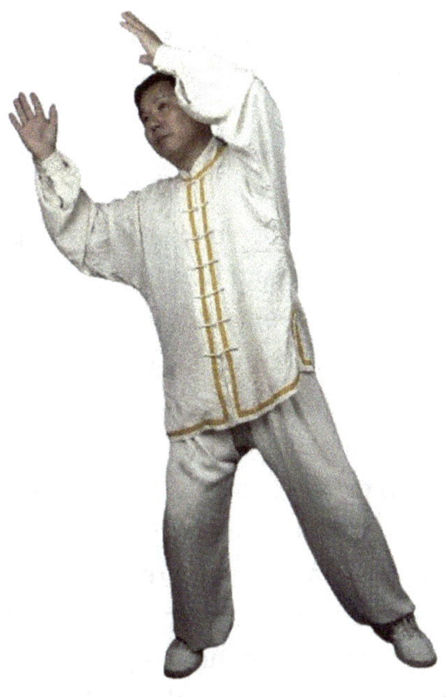

Illustration 5-8 Heavenly Dragon Waves its Tail

Just after the previous movement, the body turns left, the body's center of gravity lowers over the space between both legs to squat down, changing into a horse stance. At the same time, both hands from the upper right move downward, moving smoothly to the left and down, stopping at both sides of the chest Hua Gai acupuncture points, the fingertips are forward and up, the little fingers are kept close. Also at the same time, the Dan Tian sinks inward, slowly breathe in, using one breath in to complete the previous three movements. The tip of the tongue presses against the upper palate, the teeth are slightly closed, the eyes follow the turning of the body, the intention is on the little finger Shao Ze acupuncture point, the breath travels through the hand Da Yang Xiaochang channel. (Illustration 5-8)

5) Push Down, Return to the Beginning

These movements are entirely the same as Extreme Emptiness Exercise, Blend the Elements with One Breath (see Illustration 1-8).

Main Points and Functions

In practicing Supporting Heaven Exercise, the spirit and the inner breath begin to penetrate and flow, the outer shape and the turning are correct, the movement is natural and relaxed, the whole body sways as one. When pressing upward to support heaven, the body should remain straight, use the waist as an axle, both arms bend, both palms extend as much as possible toward the front and up to press upward with the palms. Both feet cannot leave the ground, the toes grip the ground. The centers of the feet Yong Quan acupuncture points raise upward, the palms Lao Gong acupuncture points push up, the center at the crown of the head Bai Hui acupuncture point lifts upward, these three centers together use strength to raise up, causing inner breath to move upward, the body leans slightly back, extending the abdomen and setting the elbows. The movements of Supporting Heaven must be coordinated with breathing out, when one limb moves one hundred limbs wave together, when one is quiet, there is none that is not quiet. The requirement is to achieve: calm yet not drifting, neither too much nor too little.

Heavenly Dragon waves its tail left, shakes right, and squats down these three movements must be accomplished with one breath in. Breathe in then the body moves, do not breathe in then the body is still. The waist and the back are the body's masters, with regard to the health of the body and the strength of the physique both have visible and important functions. The spine, because the Du Mai travels along this path, so then the back must be aligned and relaxed, thus helping the inner breath circulate. At the same time, it is important to pay attention that the waist and abdomen do not stick out to the front, this can make the movement more complete, remove the head-heavy feet-light disadvantage common in practice of Supporting Heaven Exercise, and helps with circulating the inner breath through the back three gates. The back three gates refer to three gates and locations along the Du Mai route that the breath and blood cannot easily pass through. The back three gates are generally referred to as: the lower end of the spine Weilu gate, the Jia Ji Lulu gate (Hua Tuo's Jia Ji), and the back of the head Yu Zhen gate.

Energy and breath rise through the back three gates along the Du Mai to the crown of the head Bai Hui acupuncture point, then, move down through the Xuan Guan opening along the Ren Mai, through the tip of the tongue, sinking down, crossing the Shan Zhong, straight into the Dan Tian. This exercise mobilizes the human life potential, using the spirit and energy to connect with the physical body, using the intention and thoughts to control the animating spirit, if there is sickness to get rid of the sickness, if there is no sickness, to develop the body, gradually achieving the purpose of extending the years and prolonging life.

Practice Method:

Each time, practice 6 times or 9 times to make one set, practicing again and again in succession is fine. The extent of the movement being larger or smaller, moving higher or lower is without restriction, depending on the age of the person practicing being older or younger, whether the physical strength is greater or lesser, and the weakness or strength in the body.

Acupuncture Points 点穴 (dian xue)

Du Mai 督脉 Governing Vessel GV[who]

Ren Mai 任脉 Controlling Vessel; Conception Vessel CV[who]

Shen Feng xue 神封穴 Spirit Seal KI-23[who]

Lao Gong xue 劳宫穴 Palace of Toil PC-8[who]

Xuan Guan qiao 玄关窍 Mysterious Gate (upper Dan Tian)

Shen Ting xue 神庭穴 Spirit Court GV-24[who]

Hua Gai xue 华盖 Florid Canopy CV-20[who]

Shao Ze xue 少泽 Lesser Marsh SI-1[who]

Da Yang Xiao Chang jing 太阳小肠经 Greater Yang Small Intestine Channel

Yong Quan xue 涌泉穴 Bubbling Spring KC-1[who]

Bai Hui xue 百会穴 Hundred Convergences GV-20[who]

Weilu guan 尾闾关 Coccyx gate

Lulu guan 辘轳关 Winch gate

Yu Zhen 玉枕 Jade Pillow BK-9[who]

Shan Zhong 膻中 (middle Dan Tian)

Set 6 Both Appear Exercise

Both Appear Exercise method distinguishes yin and yang,
I forget myself and the breath, energy, and spirit are perfected.
Dan breath seems to turn in the South,
energy and breath extend all the way to the North Star.

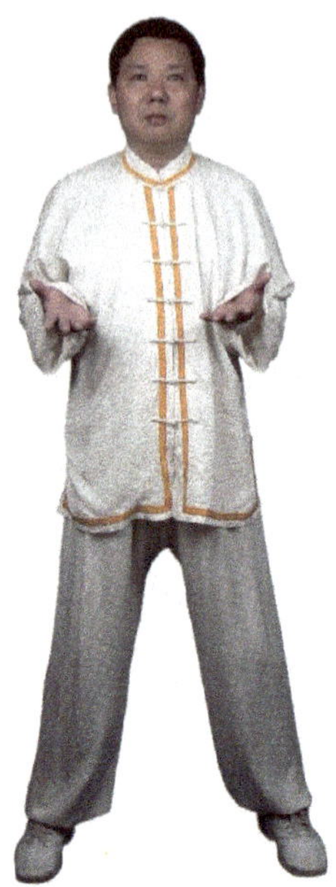

Illustration 6-1 Yin and Yang Combine with Each Other

1) Preparation

These movement methods are exactly the same as for Extreme Emptiness Exercise, Preparation Postures. (see Illustrations 1-1, 1-2, 1-3, 1-4)

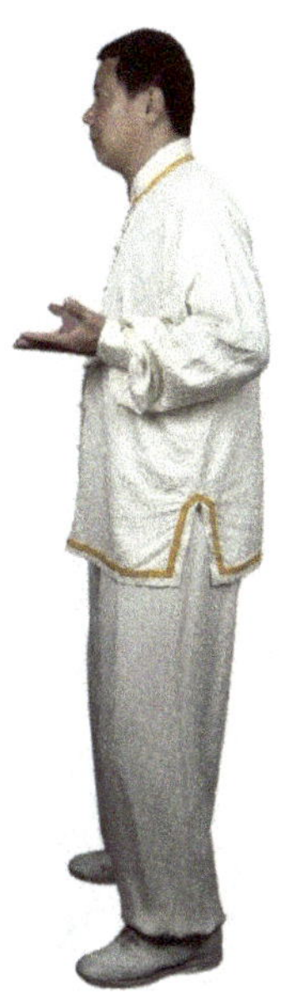

Illustration 6-2 Yin and Yang Combine with Each Other

2) Yin and Yang Combine with Each Other

The previous movement pauses slightly. After circulating the breath out and in two times, both legs extend to stand naturally. At the same time, both arms revolve to the outside; both hands together turn inward and rise upward, the heels of the palms stop just below both breasts. The fingertips of both hands point front, the palms face up. At the same time, the Dan Tian sinks inward, breathe in. The tongue rises against the upper palate, the teeth are slightly closed, the eyes look to the front. (Illustrations 6-1 and 6-2)

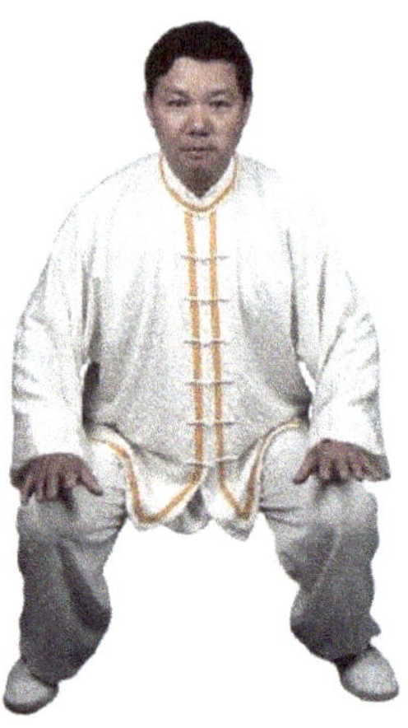

Illustration 6-3 Yin and Yang Combine with Each Other

The previous movement does not stop, the body's center of gravity lowers, both legs bend at the knees to squat down changing to a horse stance. At the same time, both arms revolve inward and both elbows hold together, the hands turn toward the front of the body in an arc shape and press down, stopping in front of the abdomen. The palms face down, the fingertips point forward. At the same time, the Dan Tian sticks outward, breathe out. The tongue rests on the lower palate; the teeth are lightly closed. The eyes look slightly downward; the intention is at the Dan Tian, the breath circulates through both the Du Mai and the Ren Mai. (Illustration 6-3)

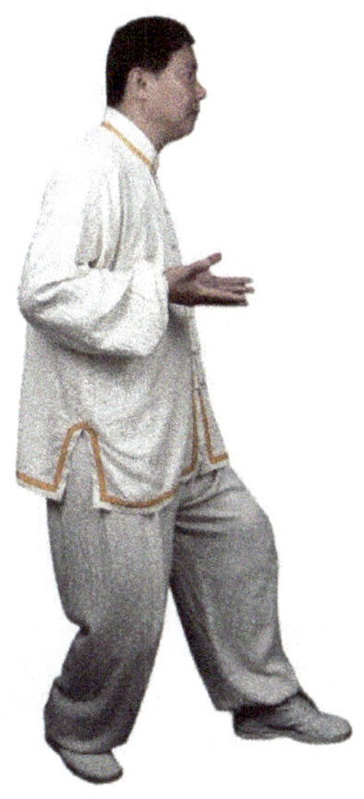

Illustration 6-4 Both Appear Left Posture

3) Both Appear Left Posture

The previous movement pauses slightly, the body's center of gravity shifts right. The body turns left 90 degrees changing to a left six four stance. The left foot toes lift, the heel stays on the ground and pulls back slightly. At the same time, both arms revolve to the outside and both hands from the front of the abdomen turn upwards describing an arc and lifting from below. The fingertips are forward; the palms face up stopping below the chest Qi Men acupuncture point. Also at the same time, the Dan Tian sinks inward, breathe in. The tip of the tongue presses against the upper palate, the teeth are slightly closed. The eyes follow the body shifting, the intention is at the centers of the feet Yong Quan acupuncture points to raise the inner breath. (Illustration 6-4)

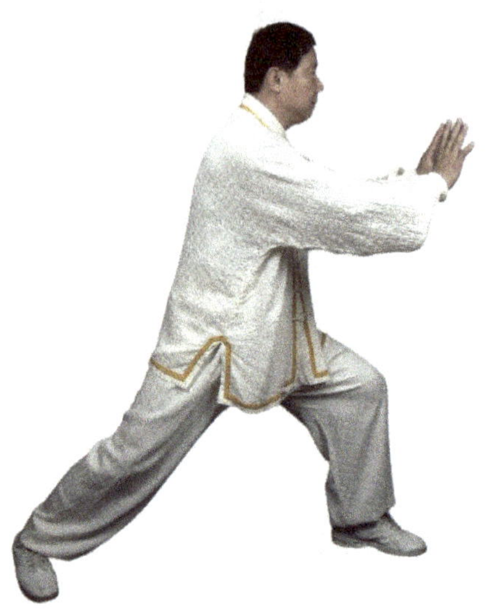

Illustration 6-5 Both Appear Left Posture

The previous movement pauses slightly, the left foot slides out half a step, the sole of the front foot presses down, the toes grip the ground. The body's center of gravity moves forward, the knee of the left leg bends slightly lower, the right leg stretches straight and presses forward changing to a left bow stance. At the same time, both arms revolve outward, both hands from below the chest push forward and up to the front in an arc shape. The fingertips are forward and up, the palms are forward and down, slightly higher than the shoulders. Also at the same time, the Dan Tian sticks outward, breathe out. The tongue rests on the lower palate, the teeth are lightly closed. The eyes look into the distance through the space between the thumbs of both hands, the intention is on the palms Lao Gong acupuncture points. The breath circulates through the hand Tai Yin Fei channel. (Illustration 6-5)

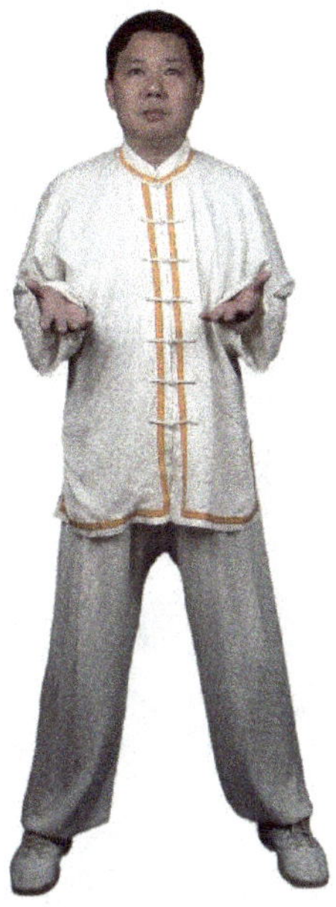

Illustration 6-6 Turn Right Small Closing

4) Turn Right Small Closing

The previous movement does not stop, the body turns right 90 degrees. After regulating the breath by breathing out and in two times two times, both legs straighten, standing naturally. At the same time, both arms revolve to the outside, both hands follow turning inward and raising upward, the heels of the palms stop just below both breasts. The fingertips are front, the palms face up. At the same time, the Dan Tian sinks inward, breathe in. The tip of the tongue presses against the upper palate, the teeth are slightly closed, the eyes look toward the front. (Illustration 6-6)

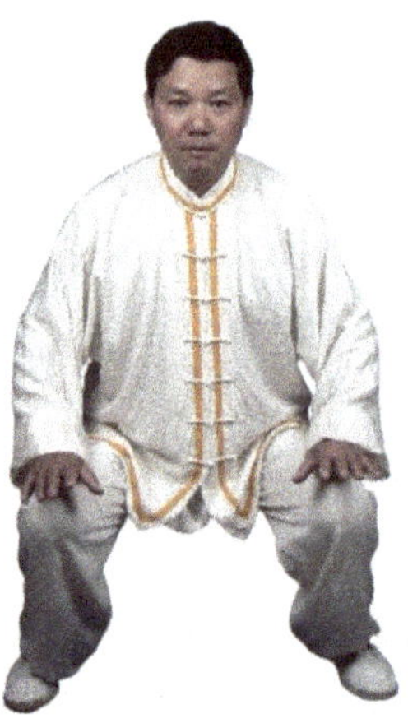

Illustration 6-7 Turn Right Small Closing

The previous movement does not stop, the body's center of gravity lowers, both legs bend at the knees to squat down changing to a horse stance. At the same time, both arms revolve inward and both elbows hold together, the hands turn toward the front of the body in an arc shape and press down, stopping in front of the abdomen. The palms face down, the fingertips point forward. At the same time, the Dan Tian sticks outward, breathe out. The tongue rests on the lower palate; the teeth are lightly closed. The eyes look slightly downward; the intention is at the Dan Tian, the breath circulates through both the Du Mai and the Ren Mai. (Illustration 6-7)

5) Both Appear Right Posture

These movement methods are entirely the same as for Both Appear Left posture, but the left and right sides are reversed (see Illustrations 6-4 and 6-5).

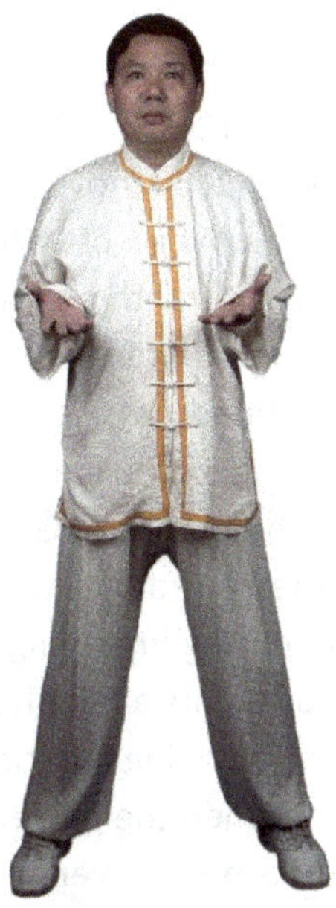

Illustration 6-8 Return to the Beginning, Closing Posture

G) Return to the Beginning, Closing Posture

The previous movement does not stop, the body turns left 90 degrees. After circulating the breath out and in two times, both legs extend to stand naturally. At the same time, both arms revolve to the outside; both hands together turn inward and rise upward, the heels of the palms stop just below both breasts. The fingertips of both hands point front, the palms face up. At the same time, the Dan Tian sinks inward, breathe in. The tongue rises against the upper palate, the teeth are slightly closed, the eyes look to the front. (Illustration 6-8)

These movements are entirely the same as Extreme Emptiness Exercise, Blend the Elements with One Breath (see Illustration 1-8).

Main Points and Functions

Both Appear Exercise can certainly and greatly transform the outward appearance of the body. Yin and yang rise and fall, movement and stillness come and go, movements are simple, then inner breath rises naturally. When breathing in, the foot three Yin Channels and the outer breath mutually connect and rise along the meridians, water and fire support each other, yin and yang are joined, then one hundred diseases can be cleared away. When practicing breathing in, the inner breath starts from the Dan Tian passes through the Hui Yin, rises through the lower Que Qiao, the Wei Lu gate, the Yao Yang gate, and the Ming Men acupuncture point. When practicing breathing out, the inner breath travels through various points along the Yin Jiao down to the Qi Hai acupuncture point, following and circulating through the tiny heavenly circle. Then, when the movements have a foundation, again practice the small heavenly circle and the large heavenly circle workmanship, then whether through one channel or a hundred channels leaving and entering will be correct.

The movements of both hands pushing down, bending the front leg, and pressing the back leg must coordinate in good order simultaneously with breathing out. The idea is to feel a warm flow, like a wheel in the tiny heavenly circle continuously turning and not stopping.

In Both Appear Exercise the outside shape of the postures must be correct and solid, inside the body the intention and inner breath have the ability to connect and circulate unobstructed, then the outer shape and strength can prosper. During practice there are also requirements for the six inside and outside connections: shoulders and hips, hands and feet, mind and intention, intention and breath, breath and strength.

The three outside connections require the movement to be round and coordinated, left and right, up and down forward and back to be together and appropriate, the posture relaxed, extended, and full; the three inside connections certainly require using the mind and the intention to mobilize the circulation of the breath and strength, where the intention goes the inner breath will travel there, joining together with the physical strength.

When the outer form moves accordingly, one can achieve a state in which the mind and spirit are joined in unity. The constitution gradually will develop increased strength, changing weakness into strength, often transforming premature aging into more youthful appearance.

Practice Method

Each time, practice 6 times or 12 times to make one set, practicing again and again in succession is fine. The extent of the movement being larger or smaller, moving higher or lower is without restriction, depending on the age of the person practicing being older or younger, whether the physical strength is greater or lesser, and the weakness or strength in the body.

Acupuncture Points 点穴 (dian xue)

Du Mai 督脉 Governing Vessel GV[who]

Ren Mai 任脉 Controlling Vessel; Conception Vessel CV[who]

Qi Men xue 期门 Cycle Gate LV-14

Yong Quan xue 涌泉穴 Bubbling Spring KC-1[who]

Lao Gong xue 劳宫穴 Palace of Toil PC-8[who]

Shou Tai Yin Fei jing 手太阴肺经 Hand's Greater Yin Lung channel LU[who]

Hui Yin 会阴 Meeting of Yin (perineum) CV-1[who]

Que Qiao 鹊桥 Bird Bridge

Weilu guan 尾闾关 Coccyx gate

Yao Yang guan 腰阳关 Lumbar Pass GV-3[who]

Ming Men xue 命门穴 Life Gate GV-4[who]

Yin Jiao 阴交 Yin Intersection CV-7[who]

Qi Hai 气海 Sea of Qi CV-6[who]

Set 7 Four Directions Exercise

Yin and Yang Both Appear gives birth to the Four Directions,

to refine the spirit continue to empty one's mind

One must know where the key to workmanship lies,

When the breath is sufficient and the spirit full,

the golden pill will mature.

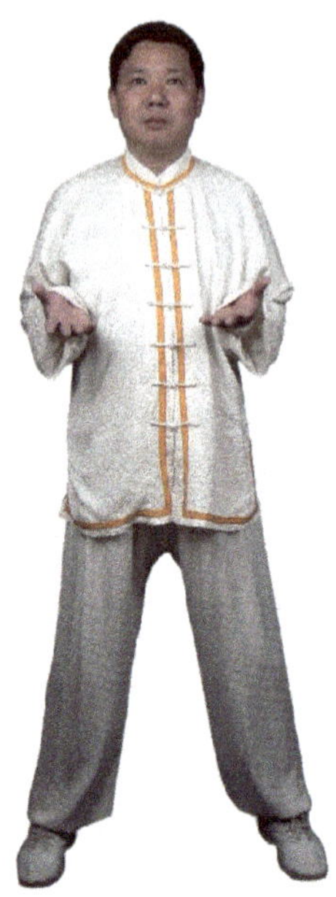

Illustration 7-1 Raise Up and Press Down

1) Preparation

These movement methods are exactly the same as for Extreme Emptiness Exercise, Preparation Postures. (see Illustrations 1-1, 1-2, 1-3, 1-4)

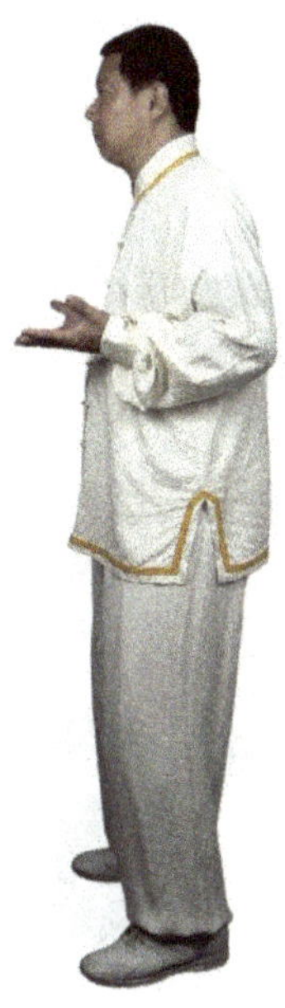

Illustration 7-2 Raise Up and Press Down

2) Raise Up and Press Down

The previous movement pauses slightly. After circulating the breath out and in two times, both legs extend to stand naturally. At the same time, both arms revolve to the outside; both hands together turn inward and rise upward, the heels of the palms stop just below both breasts. The fingertips of both hands point front, the palms face up. At the same time, the Dan Tian sinks inward, breathe in. The tongue rises against the upper palate, the teeth are slightly closed, the eyes look to the front. (Illustrations 7-1 and 7-2)

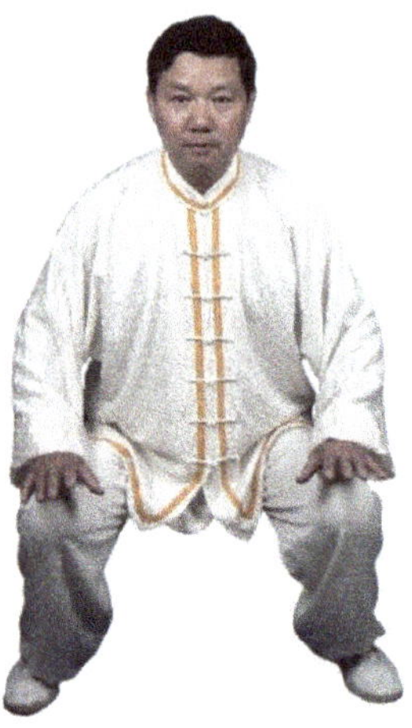

Illustration 7-3 Raise Up and Press Down

The previous movement does not stop, the body's center of gravity lowers, both legs bend at the knees to squat down changing to a horse stance. At the same time, both arms revolve inward and both elbows hold together, the hands turn toward the front of the body in an arc shape and press down, stopping in front of the abdomen. The palms face down, the fingertips point forward. At the same time, the Dan Tian sticks outward, breathe out. The tongue rests on the lower palate; the teeth are lightly closed. The eyes look slightly downward; the intention is at the Dan Tian, the breath circulates through both the Du Mai and the Ren Mai. (Illustration 7-3)

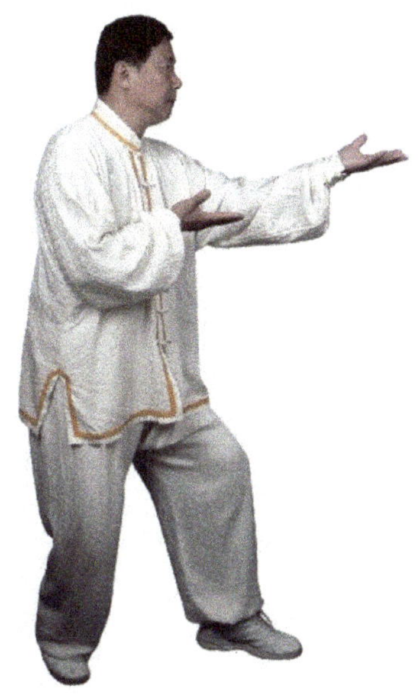

Illustration 7-4 Four Directions, Left Posture

3) Four Directions, Left Posture

The previous movement pauses slightly, the body's center of gravity slightly shifts to the right, the body turns left 90 degrees, the left heel leaves the ground and the foot pulls back to stop in front of the right foot arch changing to a left high empty step. At the same time, both arms revolve outward, both hands from the front of the abdomen up and toward the left rise up in an arc shape. The left hand is in front at the same height as the shoulder, the fingertips point front and upward, the palm faces up; the right hand stops at the inside of the left elbow joint, the fingertips point front, the palm faces up. While pressing the palms upward, the Dan Tian sinks inward, breathe in. The tongue pushes against the upper palate, the teeth are slightly closed. The eyes follow the turning of the body, the intention is on keeping the index fingers and the thumbs open. (Illustration 7-4)

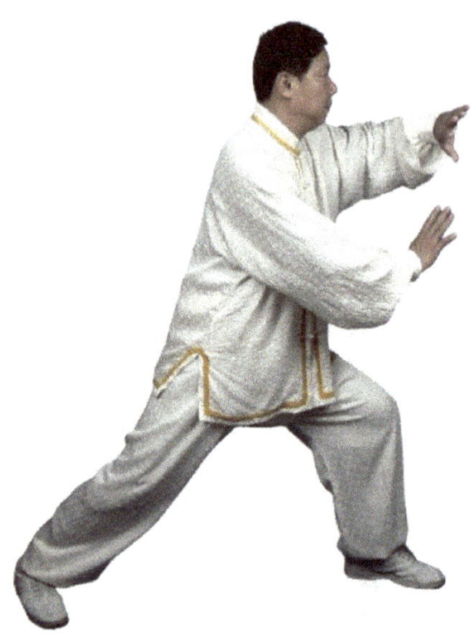

Illustration 7-5 Four Directions, Left Posture

The previous movement does not stop, the left foot steps forward a half step, the toes close inward, the left leg bends at the knee to squat down; the right leg extends and the knee straightens changing into a left bow stance. At the same time, use the waist to drive both palms, the arms revolve inward, both hands in front of the chest turn a vertical circle, then toward the left and up turning over horizontally and pushing out. The left hand fingertips point to the right, the palm faces forward at the same height as the shoulder; the right hand stops at 10 centimeters below the left palm, the fingertips point up, the palm faces forward. Also at the same time, the Dan Tian sticks outward, breathe out. The tongue rests on the lower palate, the teeth are lightly closed. The eyes look to the left and front, the intention is on the palm Lao Gong acupuncture points. (Illustration 7-5)

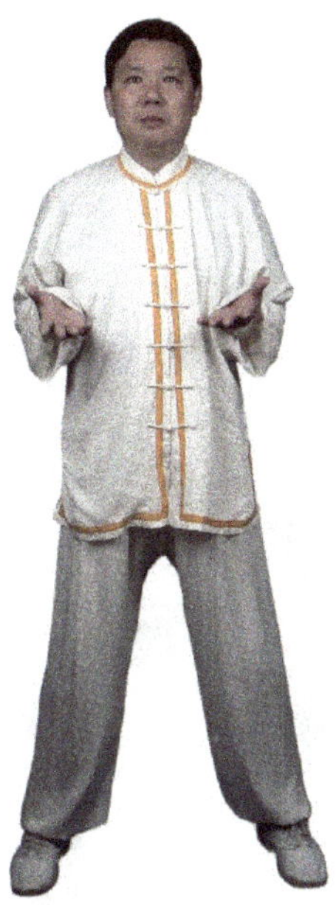

Illustration 7-6 Turn Right, Small Conclusion

4) Turn Right, Small Conclusion

The previous movement pauses slightly, the body turns right 90 degrees. After circulating the breath out and in two times, both legs extend to stand naturally. At the same time, both arms revolve to the outside; both hands together turn inward and rise upward, the heels of the palms stop just below both breasts. The fingertips of both hands point front, the palms face up. At the same time, the Dan Tian sinks inward, breathe in. The tongue rises against the upper palate, the teeth are slightly closed, the eyes look to the front. (Illustration 7-6)

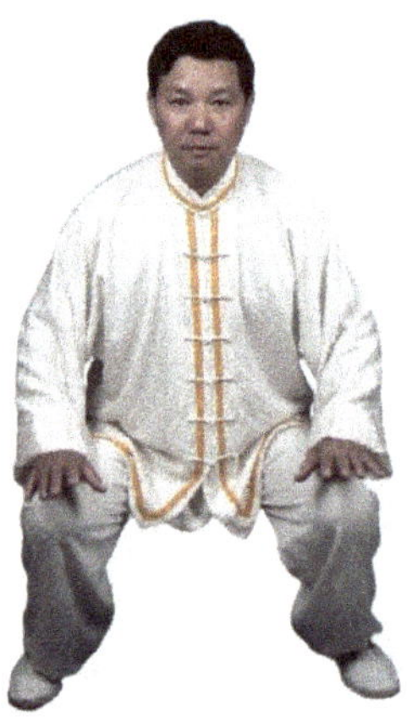

Illustration 7-7 Turn Right, Small Conclusion

The previous movement does not stop, the body's center of gravity lowers, both legs bend at the knees to squat down changing to a horse stance. At the same time, both arms revolve inward and both elbows hold together, the hands turn toward the front of the body in an arc shape and press down, stopping in front of the abdomen. The palms face down, the fingertips point forward. At the same time, the Dan Tian sticks outward, breathe out. The tongue rests on the lower palate; the teeth are lightly closed. The eyes look slightly downward; the intention is at the Dan Tian, the breath circulates through both the Du Mai and the Ren Mai. (Illustration 7-7)

5) Four Directions, Right Posture

These movement methods are entirely the same as for Both Appear Left posture, but the left and right sides are reversed (Illustrations 7-4 and 7-5)

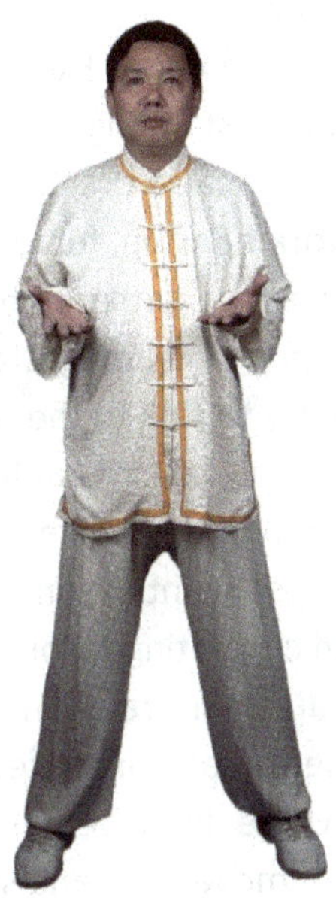

Illustration 7-8 Return to the Beginning, Closing Posture

6) Return to the Beginning, Closing Posture

The previous movement pauses slightly, the body turns left 90 degrees. After circulating the breath out and in two times, both legs extend to stand naturally. At the same time, both arms revolve to the outside; both hands together turn inward and rise upward, the heels of the palms stop just below both breasts. The fingertips of both hands point front, the palms face up. At the same time, the Dan Tian sinks inward, breathe in. The tongue rises against the upper palate, the teeth are slightly closed, the eyes look to the front. (Illustration 7-8)

These movements are entirely the same as Extreme Emptiness Exercise, Blend the Elements with One Breath (see Illustration 1-8).

Main Points and Functions

When practicing Four Directions Exercise focus on the essentials “Emptying, leading, standing strength, sink the inner breath to the Dan Tian.” This is also practiced in many other breath exercises, inner workmanship, for workmanship practitioners it is declared at the outset to be the first major requirement. Without emptying, leading, standing strength, the inner breath then is not easy to sink to the Dan Tian. In practicing China's Daoist Wudang Qigong, regard cultivating inner breath as the master, cultivating the inner breath in the shapes of the postures, just like it requires the intention and breath to pass through. The inner breath circulating through the waist supports the Chong Mai and Du Mai, inner breath in the kidney is replenished, then the inner breath circulates through the whole body, penetrating everywhere. In movement, seek stillness, in stillness, begin movement, movement and stillness give birth to each other, then the inner breath guides the changes in the postures, the uses are endless. Revolving left turning right, rising and lowering, entering forward or retreating backward, all help the person practicing to circulate inner breath smoothly, to move inner strength through the postures.

The practice of Four Directions Skill also requires practice to achieve: serious and careful, inside and outside as one. The movements of the whole body and the breathing in and out must be connected and coordinated. Pay attention to: the three centers must be combined, the three intentions must be connected, the five elements must be follow and connect. The mind is naturally relaxed, with no sense of anxiety or exertion. The three centers combine refers to the crown center Bai Hui acupuncture point to inhale downward and raise the inner breath (namely Yang Qi), the foot center Yong Quan acupuncture points breathe in and send the inner breath down (namely Yin Qi), the hand centers Lao Gong acupuncture points retract to draw in Middle Qi. So then what is above is easy to send down, what is below is easy to send up, and the middle breath is also easy to receive, then it is possible to combine all into one, return to the secret, collect in the Dan Tian. The three intentions, are the heart intention, breath intention and strength intention these three are a coherent whole.

The five elements must follow in sequence, this refers to the outer form of entering, leaving, look left, look right, and centering appearance and changes must with the body inner organs heart, liver, spleen, lungs, kidneys, the five internal organs inner breath mutually connect and flow smoothly, inner movement following the outside. Regulate the breathing, concentrate the spirit, and gather the breath, in the main and collateral channels breath flows and circulates smoothly without impediment, in a continuous cycle, the inner breath and blood can flow through the whole body, flowing and not stopping, a hundred channels flow, inside and outside connected, body and mind healthy and peaceful.

Practice Method:

Each time, practice 6 times or 9 times to make one set. Practicing again and again in succession is fine. The size of the movements, large or small, high or low is not restricted, but depends on the age or youth, the extent of physical strength, and the strength or weakness in the physique of the one who is practicing.

Acupuncture Points 点穴 (dian xue)

Du Mai 督脉 Governing Vessel GV[who]

Ren Mai 任脉 Controlling Vessel; Conception Vessel CV[who]

Chong Mai 冲脉 Thoroughfare Vessel; Penetrating Vessel PV

Bai Hui xue 百会穴 Hundred Convergences GV-20[who]

Yong Quan xue 涌泉穴 Bubbling Spring KC-1[who]

Lao Gong xue 劳宫穴 Palace of Toil PC-8[who]

Set 8 Ward Off and Pull Down Exercise

Ward Off and Pull Down Exercise methods

are positive and wonderful,

rising and lowering to circulate the breathing,

firm and soft mutually support the breath connecting to heaven,

whether amid waves or mountains,

regard them as unimportant.

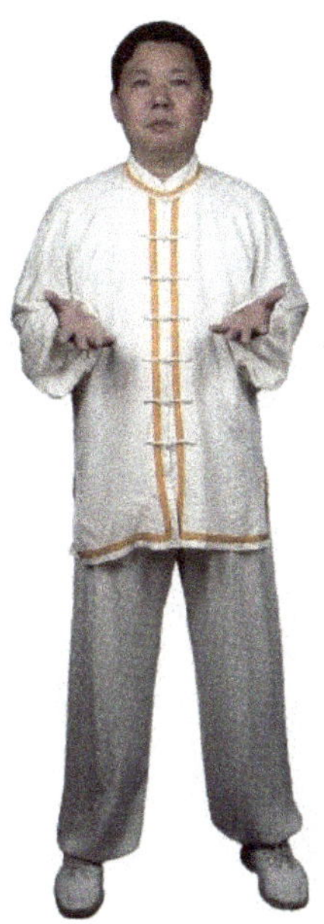

Illustration 8-1 Rise Fully, Lower Deeply

1) Preparation

These movement methods are exactly the same as for Extreme Emptiness Exercise, Preparation Postures. (see Illustrations 1-1, 1-2, 1-3, 1-4)

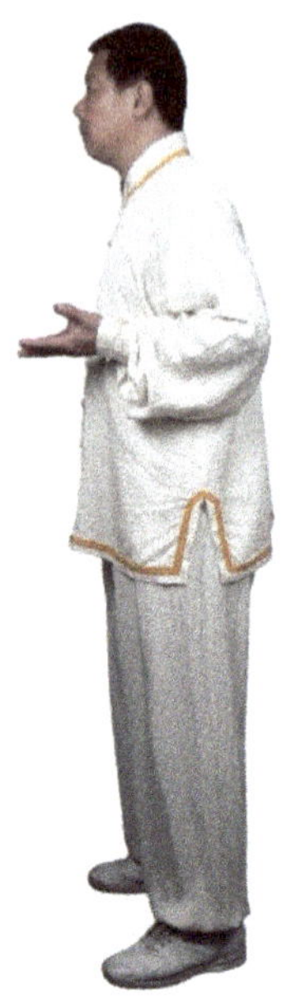

Illustration 8-2 Rise Fully, Lower Deeply

2) Rise Fully, Lower Deeply

The previous movement pauses slightly. After circulating the breath out and in two times, both legs extend to stand naturally. At the same time, both arms revolve to the outside; both hands together turn inward and rise upward, the heels of the palms stop just below both breasts. The fingertips of both hands point front, the palms face up. At the same time, the Dan Tian sinks inward, breathe in. The tongue rises against the upper palate, the teeth are slightly closed, the eyes look to the front. (Illustrations 8-1 and 8-2)

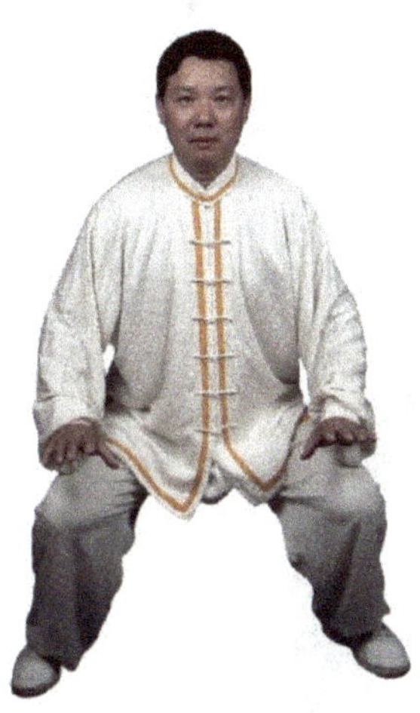

Illustration 8-3 Rise Fully, Lower Deeply

The previous movement does not stop, the body's center of gravity lowers, both legs bend at the knees to squat down changing to a horse stance. At the same time, both arms revolve inward and both elbows hold together, the hands turn toward the front of the body in an arc shape and press down, stopping in front of the abdomen. The palms face down, the fingertips point forward. At the same time, the Dan Tian sticks outward, breathe out. The tongue rests on the lower palate; the teeth are lightly closed. The eyes look slightly downward; the intention is at the Dan Tian, the breath circulates through both the Du Mai and the Ren Mai. (Illustration 8-3)

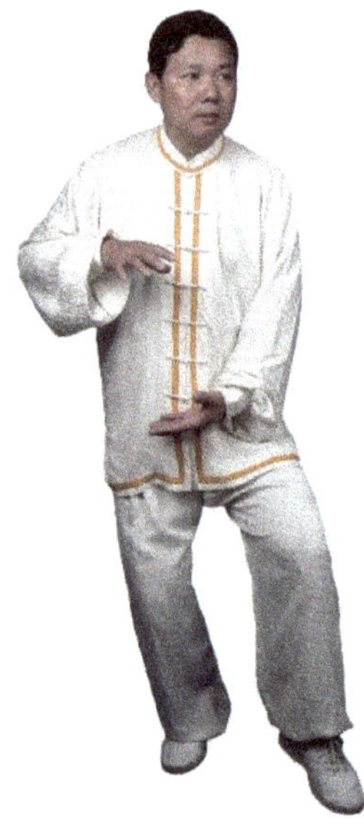

Illustration 8-4 Left Ward Off, Right Pull Down

3) Left Ward Off, Right Pull Down

The previous movement does not stop, the body's center of gravity rises, the body turns left 45 degrees standing naturally. The left arm revolves underneath, the left hand in front of the left side of the abdomen turns over, the palm faces up, the fingertips point right; the right hand rises stopping in front of the left side of the chest, fingertips point left, the palm faces down. Both hands Lao Gong acupuncture points face each other, attracting each other. Also at the same time, the Dan Tian sinks inward, breathe in. The tongue pushes against the upper palate, the teeth are slightly closed. The eyes look slightly downward, the intention is on the palm Lao Gong acupuncture points. (Illustration 8-4)

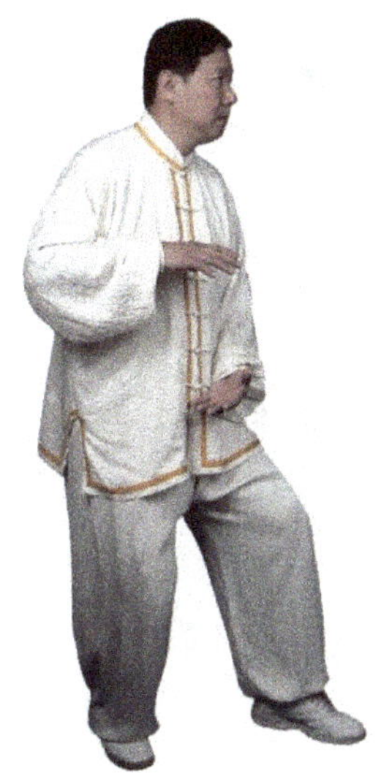

Illustration 8-5 Left Ward Off, Right Pull Down

The previous movement pauses slightly, the body's center of gravity shifts right, the body continues turning left 45 degrees, the left foot toes press the foot upward, the right heel remains on the ground changing to a left high empty stance. Also at the same time, both hands in front of the body follow the movement to hold a ball. (Illustration 8-5)

Immediately after the previous movement there is no stop, the left foot moves slightly front, the whole sole of the foot is placed on the ground, the Yong Quan acupuncture point rises, the left leg bends at the knee to half squat; the right leg knee extends and straightens changing to a left bow stance. At the same time, the left palm rises from in front of the abdomen, using the index finger to lead the inner breath in an arc shape to the left forward and upward to "ward off," at the same height as the shoulder.

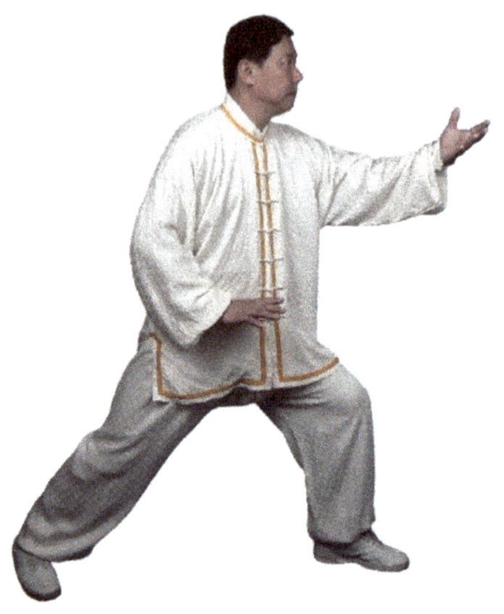

Illustration 8-6 Left Ward Off, Right Pull Down

The index finger faces the left front, the palm faces up, the breath circulates through the hand's Yang Ming Da Chang channel; the right hand from the front of the chest pulls down at an angle to right and down, stopping at the right side of the abdomen beside the Shuidao acupuncture point, the breath circulates through the foot's Yang Ming Wei channel. At the same time, the Dan Tian sticks outward, breathe out. The tongue rests on the lower palate, the teeth are lightly closed. The eyes look to the left front, the intention is on both hands index finger Shang Yang acupuncture points, both hands separate like pulling a silk thread. (Illustration 8-6)

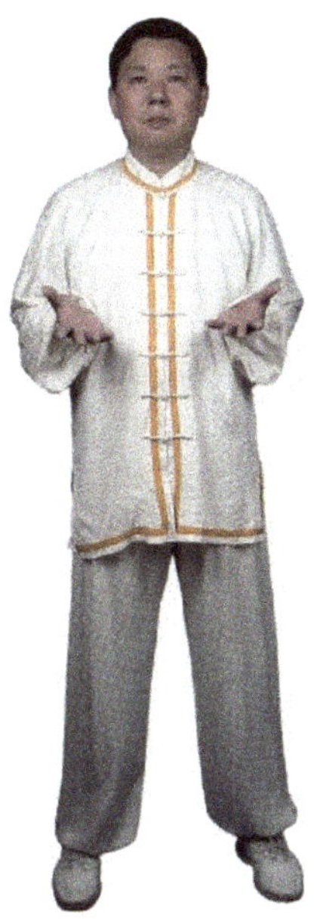

Illustration 8-7 Turn Right Combine the Breath

4) Turn Right Combine the Breath

The previous movement pauses slightly, the body turns right 90 degrees. After circulating the breath out and in two times, both legs extend to stand naturally. At the same time, both arms revolve to the outside; both hands together turn inward and rise upward, the heels of the palms stop just below both breasts. The fingertips of both hands point front, the palms face up. At the same time, the Dan Tian sinks inward, breathe in. The tongue rises against the upper palate, the teeth are slightly closed, the eyes look to the front. (Illustration 8-7)

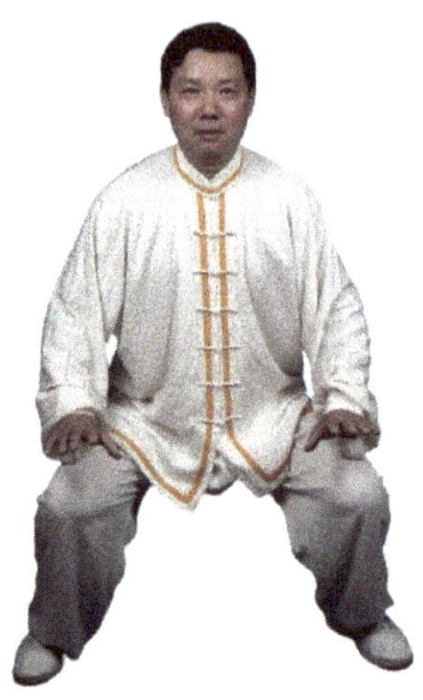

Illustration 8-8 Turn Right Combine the Breath

The previous movement does not stop, the body's center of gravity lowers, both legs bend at the knees to squat down changing to a horse stance. At the same time, both arms revolve inward and both elbows hold together, the hands turn toward the front of the body in an arc shape and press down, stopping in front of the abdomen. The palms face down, the fingertips point forward. At the same time, the Dan Tian sticks outward, breathe out. The tongue rests on the lower palate; the teeth are lightly closed. The eyes look slightly downward; the intention is at the Dan Tian, the breath circulates through both the Du Mai and the Ren Mai. (Illustration 8-8)

5) Right Ward Off, Left Pull Down

These movement methods are entirely the same as for Both Appear Left posture, but the left and right sides are reversed (see Illustrations 8-4, 8-5, and *8-6).*

6) Return the Body Restoring Posture

This movement method is entirely the same as for Pushing the Mountain Extremely Empty Initially (see Illustration 2-1). The previous movement does not stop, the next movement method is entirely the same as Extreme Emptiness Exercise, Blend the Elements with one breath (see Illustration 1-8).

Main Points and Functions

When practicing, it is important to pay attention during practice of "ward off and pull down" to the inner breath circulation through the main and collateral channels. First, the intention moves, then the intention leads the inner breath, flowing through the Dai Mai and returning through the Chong Mai, up and down, the inner breath and blood flowing together. These movements are wide open and closed, rising is yang lowering is yin. After both hands hold a ball in front of the abdomen, the index fingers pull and tug against each other. When sending out ward off, the shoulders relax, the elbows sink down, the wrist holds, the arms round, the five fingers naturally separate, the index finger lifts outward, the other four fingers slightly close to the inside, the palm must be contained, the inner breath passes through the tips of the index fingers. During "pull down," the wrist joint must sit down, the index finger remains raised, the other four fingers grab downward very much the same as grabbing at a gourd in the water, the whole movement is inseparable, connected, and not drifting.

When breathing in, try to do it without sound, continuously unbroken, without shape and without outward appearance, the breath cannot be sluggish unsmooth gasping. A person uses inner breath as a foundation, uses mind as the root, uses intention as the master. Heaven cannot be without yin and yang, people cannot be without breathing.

With one breath out a hundred channels all open, with one breath in, a hundred channels all combine. Heaven and earth require yin and yang, true breath must circulate, and none can be separated from breathing in and breathing out. When practicing, the breathing in and breathing out must in all ways be natural, conform with the regulations for practice. Moving the inner breath the regulations of course are “light out slow in,” breathing in and out mainly through the nose. In order for the strength to be vigorous and the inner breath smooth, the heart to be empty and the belly is full, naturally practice to achieve perfection.

Practice Method:

Each time, practice 6 times or 12 times to make one set, practicing again and again in succession is fine. The extent of the movement being larger or smaller, moving higher or lower is without restriction, depending on the age of the person practicing being older or younger, whether the physical strength is greater or lesser, and the weakness or strength in the body.

Acupuncture Points 点穴 (dian xue)

Du Mai 督脉 Governing Vessel GV[who]

Ren Mai 任脉 Controlling Vessel; Conception Vessel CV[who]

Lao Gong xue 劳宫穴 Palace of Toil PC-8[who]

Yong Quan xue 涌泉穴 Bubbling Spring KC-1[who]

Shou Yang Ming Dachang jing 手阳明大肠经 Hand's Yang Brightness Large Intestine channel LI[who]

Shuidao xue 水道穴 Waterway ST-28[who]

Zu Yang Ming Wei Jing 足阳明胃经 Foot's Yang Brightness Stomach channel ST[who]

Shang Yang xue 商阳穴 Shang Yang LI-1[who]

Dai Mai 带脉 Girdling Vessel GIV, GB-26[who]

Chong Mai 冲脉 Thoroughfare Vessel; Penetrating Vessel PV

Set 9 Pipa Exercise

Three times play the pipa[18] *on each side,*

yin and yang naturally change within.

Intention breath is the monarch

the bones and flesh are subjects,

heaven's energy and earth's sprit nourish the golden pill.

---

[18] 琵琶 pipa - a Chinese stringed musical instrument similar to the English lute.

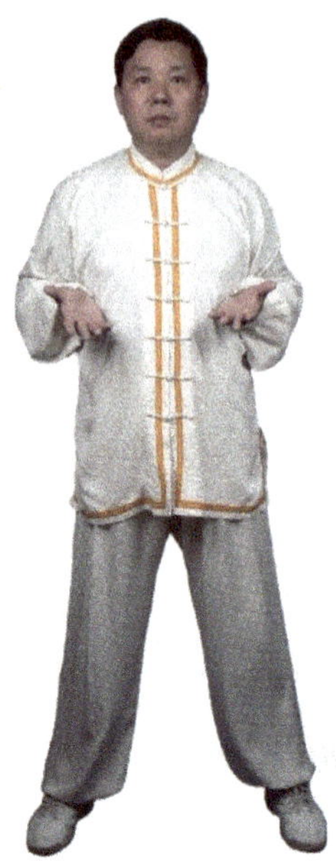

Illustration 9-1 Regulate the Breath Up and Down

1) Preparation

These movement methods are exactly the same as for Extreme Emptiness Exercise, Preparation Postures. (see Illustrations 1-1, 1-2, 1-3, 1-4)

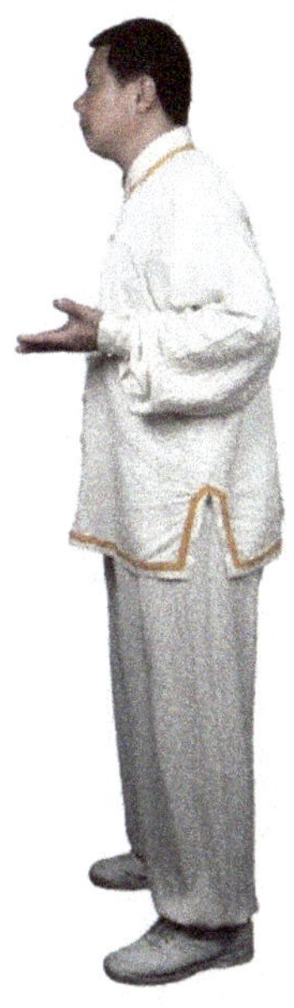

Illustration 9-2 Regulate the Breath Up and Down

2) Regulate the Breath Up and Down

The previous movement pauses slightly. After circulating the breath out and in two times, both legs extend to stand naturally. At the same time, both arms revolve to the outside; both hands together turn inward and rise upward, the heels of the palms stop just below both breasts. The fingertips of both hands point front, the palms face up. At the same time, the Dan Tian sinks inward, breathe in. The tongue rises against the upper palate, the teeth are slightly closed, the eyes look to the front. (Illustrations 9-1 and 9-2)

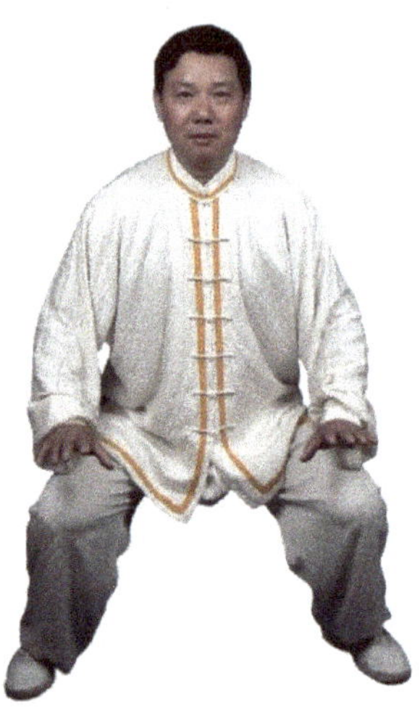

Illustration 9-3 Regulate the Breath Up and Down

The previous movement does not stop, the body's center of gravity lowers, both legs bend at the knees to squat down changing to a horse stance. At the same time, both arms revolve inward and both elbows hold together, the hands turn toward the front of the body in an arc shape and press down, stopping in front of the abdomen. The palms face down, the fingertips point forward. At the same time, the Dan Tian sticks outward, breathe out. The tongue rests on the lower palate; the teeth are lightly closed. The eyes look slightly downward; the intention is at the Dan Tian, the breath circulates through both the Du Mai and the Ren Mai. (Illustration 9-3)

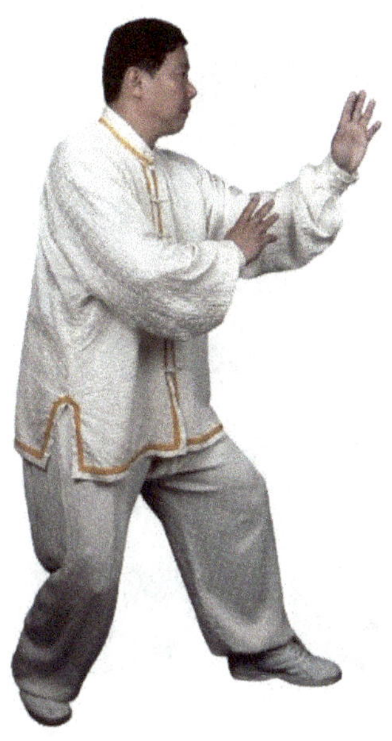

Illustration 9-4 Pipa Left Posture

3) Pipa Left Posture

The previous movement pauses slightly, the body's center of gravity shifts right, the body turns left 90 degrees, the left foot toes press upward changing to a left high empty stance. At the same time, both hands with vertical palms drill out and up to the left. The left palm is slightly higher than the shoulder, the fingertips point front, the palm faces right; the right palm stops at the inside of the left elbow joint, the fingertips point up, the palm faces left. Also at the same time, the Dan Tian turns inward and sinks in, breathe in. The tongue rises against the upper palate, the teeth are slightly closed. The eyes follow the motion of the left hand fingers, the intention is at the crown of the head Bai Hui acupuncture point. (Illustration 9-4)

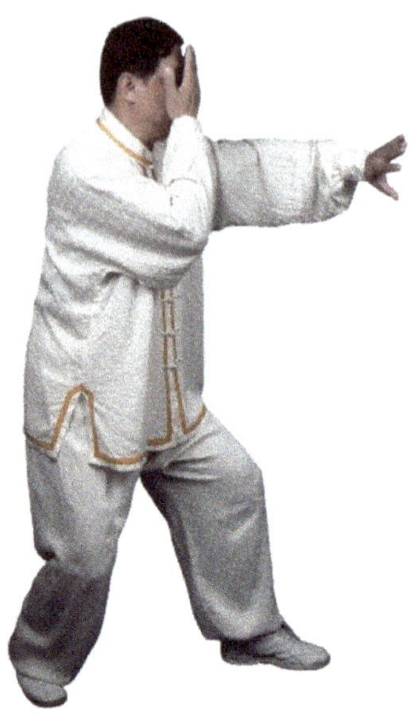

Illustration 9-5 Pipa Left Posture

The previous movement does not stop, the body turns slightly toward the left, the left arm revolves outward, the left palm circles back and turns, the fingertips point up, the center of the palm Lao Gong acupuncture point is in front of the left side Si Bai acupuncture point; the right arm revolves inward, the right palm fingers use strength in turning outward to strike,[19] the fingertips point left, the palm faces front. (Illustration 9-5)

[19] 弹拨 tanbo - to pluck or strike; to play a musical instrument. The pipa is played by plucking its strings.

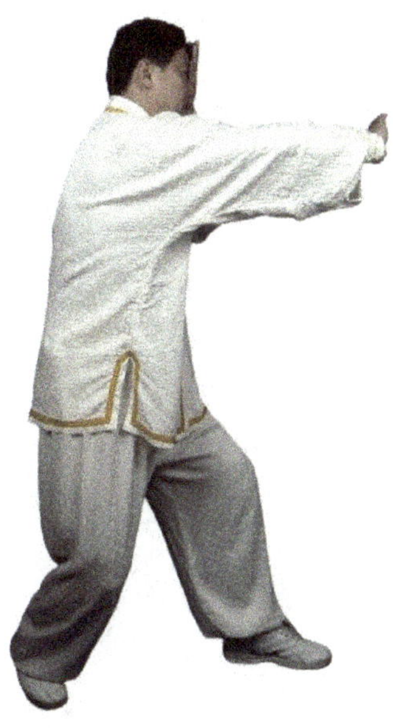

Illustration 9-6 Pipa Left Posture

Just after the previous movement, the body turns slightly to the right, the right arm revolves outward, the right palm circles back and turns, the fingertips face up, the center of the palm Lao Gong acupuncture point is in front of the right side Si Bai acupuncture point; the left arm revolves inward; the fingers of the left palm use strength in turning outward to strike, the fingertips face right, the center of the palm faces front. Also at the same time, the Dan Tian sticks outward, gradually breathe out. The tongue rests on the lower palate, the teeth are lightly closed. The eyes follow the movement of the hands, the intention is on the Lao Gong acupuncture point facing the Si Bai extending warm breath. (Illustration 9-6)

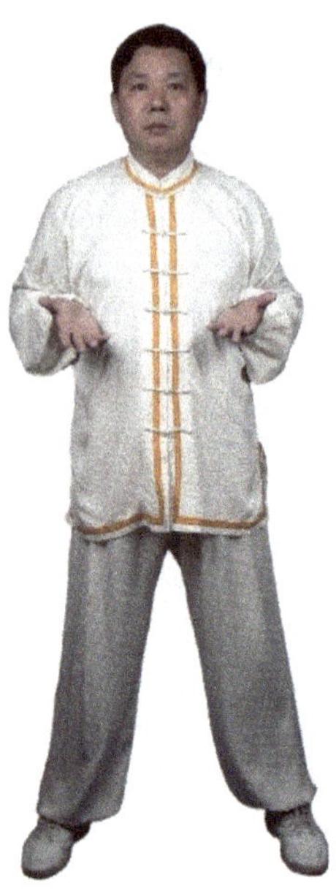

Illustration 9-7 Turn Right, Connect the Breath

4) Turn Right, Connect the Breath

The previous movement pauses slightly, the body turns to the right 90 degrees. After circulating the breath out and in two times, both legs extend to stand naturally. At the same time, both arms revolve to the outside; both hands together turn inward and rise upward, the heels of the palms stop just below both breasts. The fingertips of both hands point front, the palms face up. At the same time, the Dan Tian sinks inward, breathe in. The tongue rises against the upper palate, the teeth are slightly closed, the eyes look to the front. (Illustration 9-7)

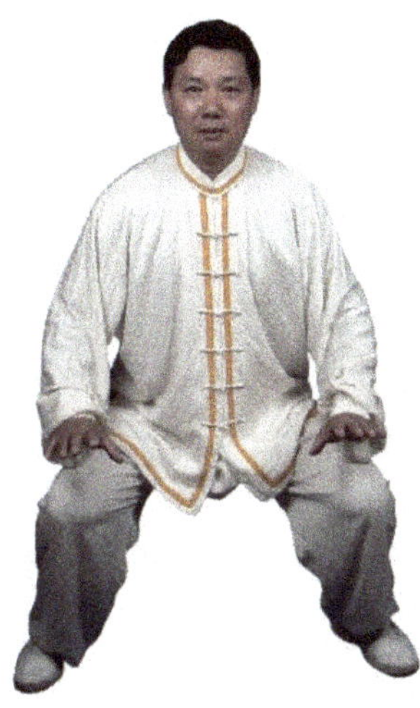

Illustration 9-8 Turn Right, Connect the Breath

The previous movement does not stop, the body's center of gravity lowers, both legs bend at the knees to squat down changing to a horse stance. At the same time, both arms revolve inward and both elbows hold together, the hands turn toward the front of the body in an arc shape and press down, stopping in front of the abdomen. The palms face down, the fingertips point forward. At the same time, the Dan Tian sticks outward, breathe out. The tongue rests on the lower palate; the teeth are lightly closed. The eyes look slightly downward; the intention is at the Dan Tian, the breath circulates through both the Du Mai and the Ren Mai. (Illustration 9-8)

5) Pipa Right Posture

These movement methods are entirely the same as for Pipa Left posture, but the left and right sides are reversed (see Illustrations 9-4, 9-5, and 9-6).

6) Turn the Body, Return to the Beginning

This movement method is entirely the same as for Pushing the Mountain Extremely Empty Initially (see Illustration 2-1). The previous movement does not stop, the next movement method is entirely the same as Extreme Emptiness Exercise, Blend the Elements with one breath (see Illustration 1-8).

Main Points and Functions

In practicing Pipa Skill, the major point is to nourish the kidneys and strengthen the kidneys. The kidneys support the bones, the bones create marrow, while "the brain is the sea of marrow." So then, when kidney energy is abundant, naturally energy and strength will be plentiful, the thoughts quick and agile, the memory strong, and the muscles and bones sturdy.

In this exercise, the movements are not only comfortable and soft, but also open and extended. In the correct way of considering relaxing, the whole body muscles, limbs, bones, blood, all must expand and contract. Afterward, hard and soft must be balanced, the whole body up and down forms changing as a whole body, well-connected and coordinated, in movement there is stillness, in stillness there is movement.

In practicing Pipa Skill, it is also important to pay attention to avoiding the "3 restrictions" namely, the shape of the body restriction, thought restriction, and breathing restriction. When the body is naturally relaxed, then it cannot be stiff and inflexible, nor can it be weak and without strength, to achieve relaxed but not slack, the whole form has an inner vigor.

The thoughts must be relaxed and light, living and breathing, holding but not holding, not expecting and not trying, it cannot be forced. The breathing should be natural and leisurely, slow and continuous, neither holding the breath nor forcing the breath. These three points run through the whole process of practice. The energy and breath must circulate and flow through the main and collateral channels in the whole body, with the movements both must combine. In breathing out push out, on breathing in pull back. After circulating the breath each time, there is also a "return to emptiness" and a requirement to collect the workmanship at the lower Dan Tian Qi Hai acupuncture point. In this way, over time, a long period, with painstaking practice, the inner energy and breath circulate will become more and more smooth, the circulation of the inner breath becomes greater and greater, the inner breath body has the maximum effect on the human body.

When inner breath increases there is life, when inner breath decreases there is death. A person who wants to live a long live, must cherish breathing, respect the inner spirit nuances, respect the energy (earlier heaven energy and later heaven energy). When energy, breath, spirit, are abundant then one can achieve a relaxed face, brilliant eyes, clear hearing, full of energy and spirit, the expression graceful.

Practice Method:

Each time, practice 6 times or 12 times to make one set, practicing again and again in succession is fine. The extent of the movement being larger or smaller, moving higher or lower is without restriction, depending on the age of the person practicing being older or younger, whether the physical strength is greater or lesser, and the weakness or strength in the body.

Acupuncture Points 点穴 (dian xue)

Du Mai 督脉 Governing Vessel GV[who]

Ren Mai 任脉 Controlling Vessel; Conception Vessel CV[who]

Lao Gong xue 劳宫穴 Palace of Toil PC-8[who]

Bai Hui xue 百会穴 Hundred Convergences GV-20[who]

Si Bai xue 四白穴 Four Whites ST-2[who]

Qi Hai 气海 Sea of Qi CV-6[who]

Set 10 Shaking the Tail Feathers Exercise

Transport the breath to gather and converge in the Dan Tian

In shaking feathers with both wings the intention flows outward.

To understand the mystery

raise the anus, heels, breath is the true teaching.

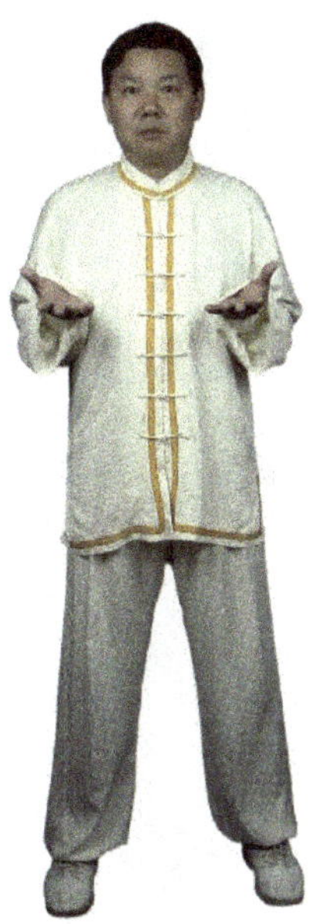

Illustration 10-1 Regulate the Breath Above and Below

1) Preparation

These movement methods are exactly the same as for Extreme Emptiness Exercise, Preparation Postures. (see Illustrations 1-1, 1-2, 1-3, 1-4)

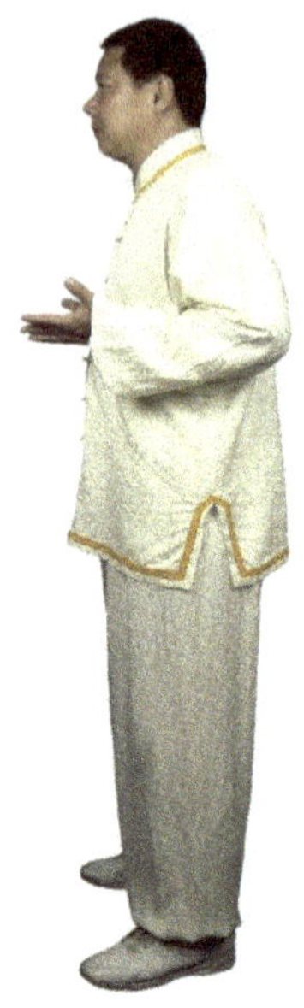

Illustration 10-2 Regulate the Breath Above and Below

2) Regulate the Breath Above and Below

The previous movement pauses slightly. After circulating the breath out and in two times, both legs extend to stand naturally. At the same time, both arms revolve to the outside; both hands together turn inward and rise upward, the heels of the palms stop just below both breasts. The fingertips of both hands point front, the palms face up. At the same time, the Dan Tian sinks inward, breathe in. The tongue rises against the upper palate, the teeth are slightly closed, the eyes look to the front. (Illustrations 10-1 and 10-2)

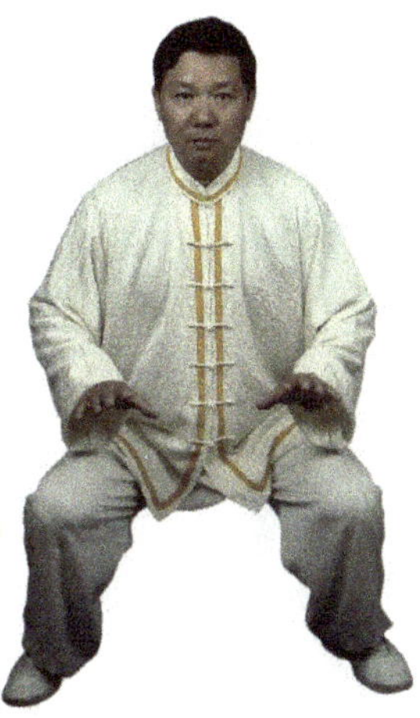

Illustration 10-3 Regulate the Breath Above and Below

The previous movement does not stop, the body's center of gravity lowers, both legs bend at the knees to squat down changing to a horse stance. At the same time, both arms revolve inward and both elbows hold together, the hands turn toward the front of the body in an arc shape and press down, stopping in front of the abdomen. The palms face down, the fingertips point forward. At the same time, the Dan Tian sticks outward, breathe out. The tongue rests on the lower palate; the teeth are lightly closed. The eyes look slightly downward; the intention is at the Dan Tian, the breath circulates through both the Du Mai and the Ren Mai. (Illustration 10-3)

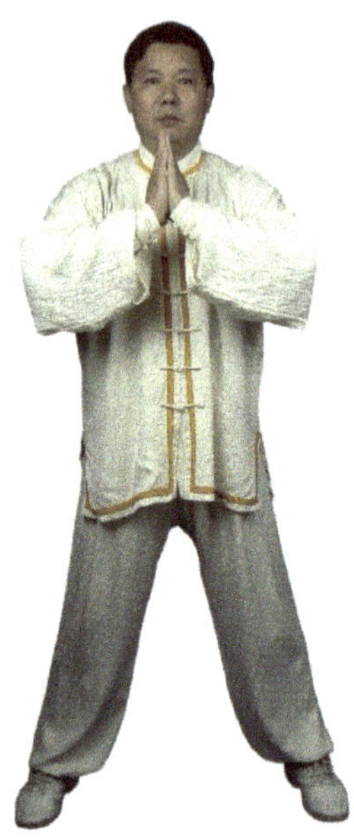

Illustration 10-4 Shaking the Tail Feathers Left Posture

3) Shaking the Tail Feathers Left Posture

The previous movement pauses slightly, both legs straighten, standing naturally straight. At the same time, both arms revolve outward and turn up, both hands rise upward, rising in front of the body, both palms come together stopping in front of the jaw. The fingertips point up, the little finger side faces front. At the same time, the Dan Tian sinks inward, breathe in. The tip of the tongue presses against the upper palate, the teeth are lightly closed. The eyes look slightly down, the intention is on the crown of the head Bai Hui acupuncture point. (Illustration 10-4)

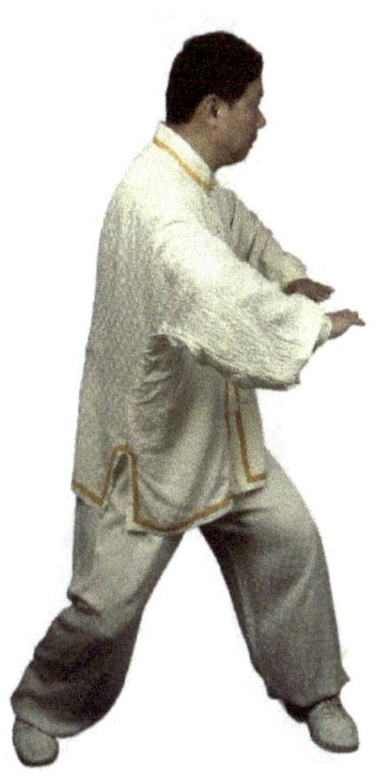

Illustration 10-5 Shaking the Tail Feathers Left Posture

The previous movement does not stop, the body turns left 90 degrees, the center of gravity is front six back four, resulting in a left six four stance. At the same time, both arms revolve inward, the hands separate in front of the chest to the side of the body turn over and open, horizontally shaking, pausing slightly at the hips. The fingertips point down obliquely, the palms face down, the little finger is toward the front of the body. Also at the same time, the Dan Tian sticks outward, breathe out. The tongue rests on the lower palate, the teeth are slightly closed. The eyes look down to the left, the intention is on the left little finger Shao Chong acupuncture point. (Illustration 10-5)

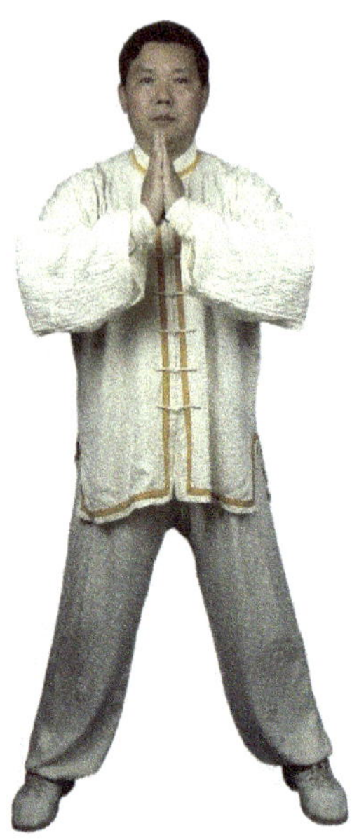

Illustration 10-6 Horse Stance, Split Right

4) Horse Stance, Split Right[20]

The previous movement does not stop, the body turns left 90 degrees, facing south and standing straight. Both arms revolve outward and turn up, both hands rise upward, rising in front of the body, both palms come together stopping in front of the jaw. The fingertips point up, the little finger side faces front. At the same time, the Dan Tian sinks inward, breathe in. The tip of the tongue presses against the upper palate, the teeth are lightly closed. The eyes follow the body movement, the intention is on the palm Lao Gong acupuncture points mutually attracting each other. (Illustration 10-6)

[20] 劈 (pi) chop, split downward

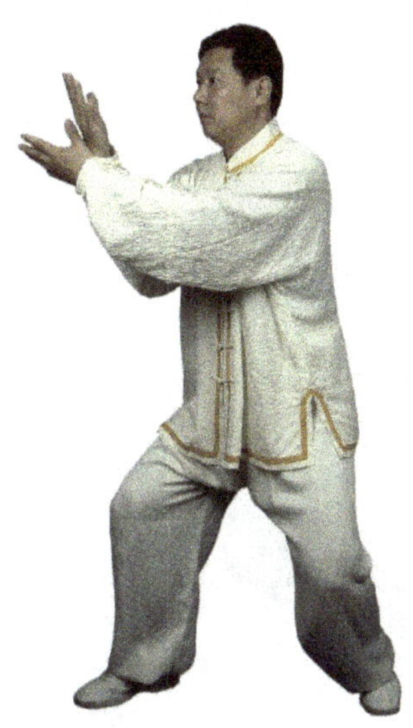

Illustration 10-7 Horse Stance, Split Right

The previous movement pauses slightly, the body slightly turns right, both legs bend at the knees changing into a horse stance. The body leans slightly toward the front, both arms revolve outward, both hands from the sides of the body rise up, rising to the front in an arc shape, the left hand fingertips point forward and up, the palm faces up; the right hand stops above the left wrist Wan Mai gate. The fingertips point to the left front, the palms face up. At the same time, the Dan Tian sinks inward, breathe in. The tongue rises against the upper palate, the teeth are slightly closed. The eyes look forward and down, the intention is on raising the foot center Yong Quan acupuncture point. (Illustration 10-7)

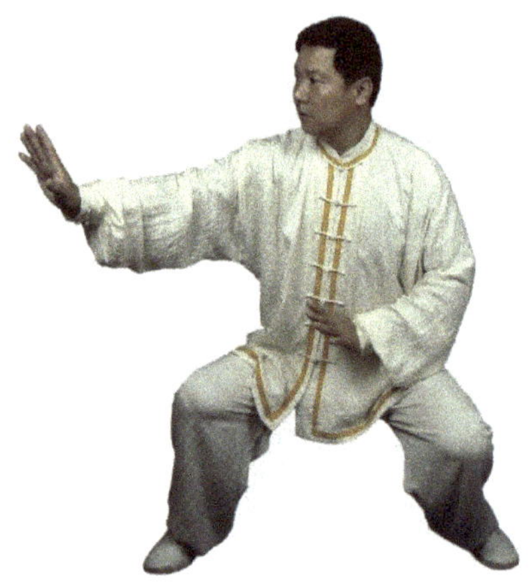

Illustration 10-8 Horse Stance, Split Right

The previous movement does not stop, the body continues turning to the right 135 degrees, the body's center of gravity sinks down. At the same time, the outside edge of the right hand uses strength to split down to the lower right front, the same height as the middle Dan Tian Shan Zhong acupuncture point, the fingertips point up to the front, the palm faces forward and down; the left hand revolves inward and presses down, stopping in front of the abdomen, the thumb joint is just above the navel, the palm faces down, the index finger is raised, mirroring the right hand index finger. When chopping with the palm, the Dan Tian sticks outward, breathe out. The tongue rests on the lower palate, the teeth are lightly closed. The eyes look at the right hand fingers, the intention is on the thumb's Shao Shang acupuncture point, the breath travels along the hand Tai Yin Fei channel. (Illustration 10-8)

5) Shaking the Tail Feathers Right Posture

These movement methods are entirely the same as for Shaking the Tail Feathers Left posture, but the left and right sides are reversed (see Illustrations 10-4, 10-5)

6) Horse Stance, Left Chop

The movement methods are exactly the same as Horse Stance, Right Chop, except that the movement is toward the other side. (see Illustrations 10-6, 10-7, 10-8)

7) Turn the Body, Go Back to the Beginning

This movement method is entirely the same as for Pushing the Mountain Extremely Empty Initially (see Illustration 2-1). The previous movement does not stop, the next movement method is entirely the same as Extreme Emptiness Exercise, Blend the Elements with one breath (see Illustration 1-8).

Main Points and Functions

Throughout the practice of Shaking the Tail Feathers, firm and soft compliment each other, use the body to lead the hands, use the intention to lead the inner breath, use the inner breath to fill the body, open and connect the meridians and channels, so the inner breath and blood are evenly distributed through the whole body to every organ. While turning to Shake the Tail Feathers, generally use reverse breathing, breathe in, sink the Dan Tian inward; breathe out, extend the Dan Tian outward. This can cause the diaphragm muscle to drop lower, respiration to deepen and lengthen, lung capacity to increase, and can promote strong metabolism. The body's center of gravity sinking down, the body turning, both elbows setting open, both palms stretching open these movements must be neat and consistent. Also strive for relaxed shoulders and level hips, the elbows sink and the knees bend, the hands connect and move with the heels. There is opening and closing; first store up, then send out. The Classics say: "Shaking the tail feathers should be formless, if there is form it will be ineffective. When sending out the hands, do not use force, using force is not refined."

Yin rises yang lowers, clear and cloudy are converted into each other. Generally, beginning practitioners of Wudang Qigong, the mouth may often have phlegm, sink down empty breath, this is the required process when turbid air lowers down, clean air rises. It is normal. Phlegm must be spit out, but inside the mouth swallow the saliva together with the inhale, so it descends down to the Dan Tian. In ancient times, this was called the water of heaven, when it enters the Dan Tian it can join water and fire, brighten and smooth the heart and kidney.

The ancients called this Water from the River of Heaven, when it descends to the Dan Tian then and only then can water and fire join together, open and moisten the heart and kidneys. During practice, the thoughts must be concentrated, when distracting thoughts emerge, within the mind repeat aloud to oneself the eight methods:

1. When the mind is calm, the spirit is tranquil,
2. When the spirit is tranquil, the mind is set at ease,
3. When the mind is set at ease, it is full and still,
4. When there is fullness and stillness, there are no disturbances,
5. When there are no disturbances, the breath can circulate,
6. When the breath can circulate, one can transcend appearances,
7. When one transcends appearances, one discovers clear understanding
8. When one discovers clear understanding, then the spirit and the breath will be joined together, and ten thousand things will return to their root.

Practice Method:

Each time, practice 6 times or 12 times to make one set, practicing again and again in succession is fine. The extent of the movement being larger or smaller, moving higher or lower is without restriction, depending on the age of the person practicing being older or younger, whether the physical strength is greater or lesser, and the weakness or strength in the body.

Acupuncture Points 点穴 (dian xue)

Du Mai 督脉 Governing Vessel GV[who]

Ren Mai 任脉 Controlling Vessel; Conception Vessel CV[who]

Bai Hui xue 百会穴 Hundred Convergences GV-20[who]

Shao Chong xue 少冲穴 Lesser Thoroughfare HT-9[who]

Lao Gong xue 劳宫穴 Palace of Toil PC-8[who]

Mai Men 脉门 Vessel Gate, Lesser Thoroughfare HT-9[who]

Yong Quan xue 涌泉穴 Bubbling Spring KC-1[who]

Set 11 White Ape Presents Fruit Exercise

White Ape[21] from the Cheng Jiang offers an immortal peach,

the old monarch bestows a Golden Pill at the furnace front.

Planting melons and growing beans is not futile,

extend outward, gather inward; naturally become immortal.

---

[21] 白猿 (Bai Yuan) White Ape - aged with white hair; an immortal ape (shen hou) 神猴

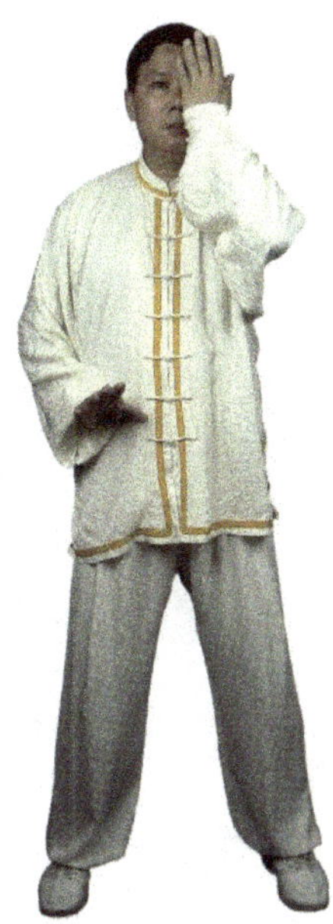

Illustration 11-1 Ape Washes its Face

1) Preparation

These movement methods are exactly the same as for Extreme Emptiness Exercise, Preparation Postures. (see Illustrations 1-1, 1-2, 1-3, 1-4)

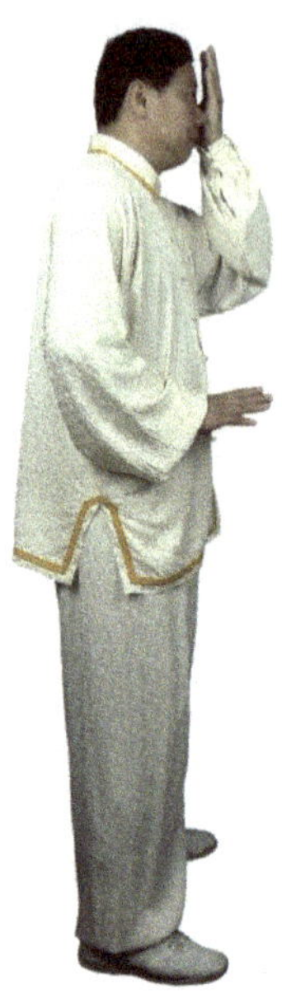

Illustration 11-2 Ape Washes its Face

2) Ape Washes its Face

The previous movement pauses slightly, the left arm revolves outward; the left hand rises from the side of the body, stopping at the outer corner of the left eye, the fingertips point up, the palm faces inward. The intention is on using the left hand Lao Gong acupuncture point to send out workmanship (fa gong) to massage downward on the left side of the face; the right hand is coordinated and rises upward, stopping outside the waist opening Dai Mai, the fingertips point front, the palm faces down. Also at the same time, the Dan Tian sinks inward, breathe in. The tongue presses against the upper palate, the teeth are lightly closed. The eyes are slightly closed, the intention is on the left palm, the breath circulates through the foot Shao Yang Dan channel. (Illustrations 11-1 and 11-2)

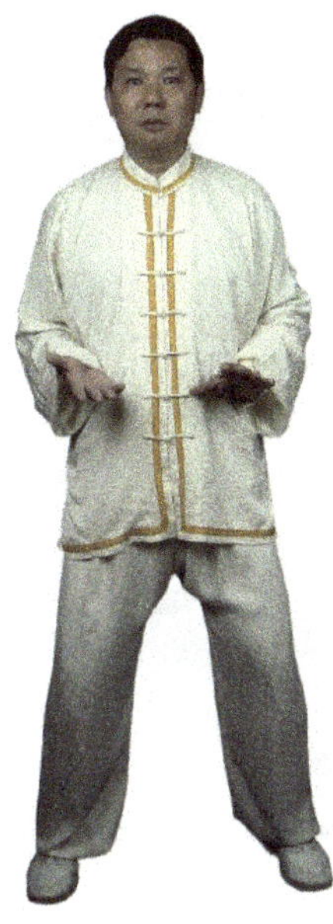

Illustration 11-3 Ape Washes its Face

The previous movement does not stop, the body's center of gravity sinks down, both legs bend at the knees to squat down changing to a horse stance. At the same time, both arms revolve inward, the left palm Lao Gong acupuncture point uses intent to press downward along the left side of the body sending out workmanship (fa gong), stopping at the waist opening Dai Mai, the fingertips point front, the palm faces down becoming a yin palm. At the same time, the right arm revolves outward, the right palm turns over changing into a yang palm and stopping at the waist, the fingertips point front, the palm faces up. At the same time, the Dan Tian sticks outward, breathe out. The tongue rests on the lower palate, the teeth are lightly closed. The eyes look forward, the intention is on the Dan Tian, the inner breath circulates through the Dai Mai. (Illustration 11-3)

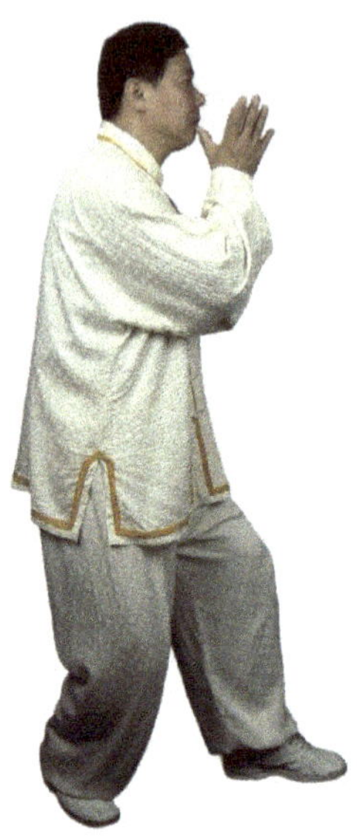

Illustration 11-4 Offering Fruit Left Posture

3) Offering Fruit Left Posture

The previous movement pauses slightly, the body's center of gravity shifts to the right leg, the body turns left 90 degrees. The left toes press upward, the right heel remains on the ground changing to a left high empty stance. Both hands from the waist toward the face arc upward, like holding something. The heels of the palms rest against each other, the fingertips are slanted upward, the thumbs of both hands are placed against the lower jaw Cheng Jiang acupuncture point. At the same time, the Dan Tian sinks inward, breathe in. The tongue rises against the upper palate, the teeth are slightly closed. The eyes follow the movement of the body, the intention is on the Yong Quan acupuncture point, the breath circulates through the hand Tai Yin Fei channel. (Illustration 11-4)

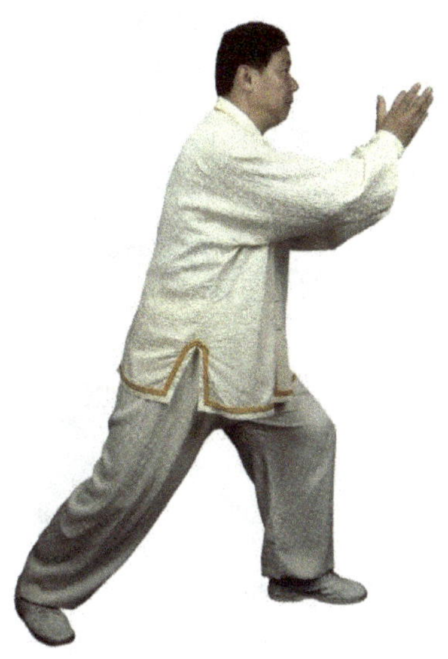

Illustration 11-5 Offering Fruit Left Posture

The previous movement does not stop, the left foot steps out half a step to the front, the whole foot presses against the ground; the left leg bends at the knee to squat; the right leg extends straight changing to a left bow stance. At the same time, both hands extend upward from outside the Cheng Jiang acupuncture point, to the left front pushing out in an arc shape, both arms straighten, pausing at the height of the eyes. The five fingers naturally open, the tiger's mouth[22] maintains a circle, the tips of the thumbs point up, the remaining four fingers point front. Also at the same time, the Dan Tian sticks outward, breathe out. The tongue rests on the lower palate, the teeth are slightly closed. The eyes follow the hands and look up, the intention is on the palm Lao Gong acupuncture points, the breath circulates through the hand Jue Yin Xinbao channel. (Illustration 11-5)

---

[22] 虎口 (hu kou) between the thumb and the index finger of the hand

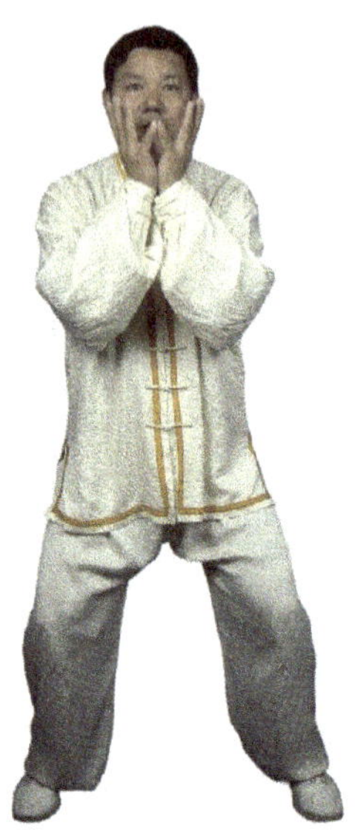

Illustration 11-6 Receive the Fruit, Collect Inside

4) Receive the Fruit, Collect Inside

The previous movement pauses slightly, the body turns right 90 degrees, the left foot slightly pulls back, the body center of gravity rises, naturally straight. At the same time, both palms return to their previous position, both hands hold a fruit and stop below the jaw. The outer side of the little finger faces front, the heels of the palms draw close stopping at the Yu Tang acupuncture point. At the same time, the Dan Tian sinks inward, breathe in. The tongue rises against the upper palate, the teeth are slightly closed. The eyes look down slightly, the intention is on the Xuan Guan opening. (Illustration 11-6)

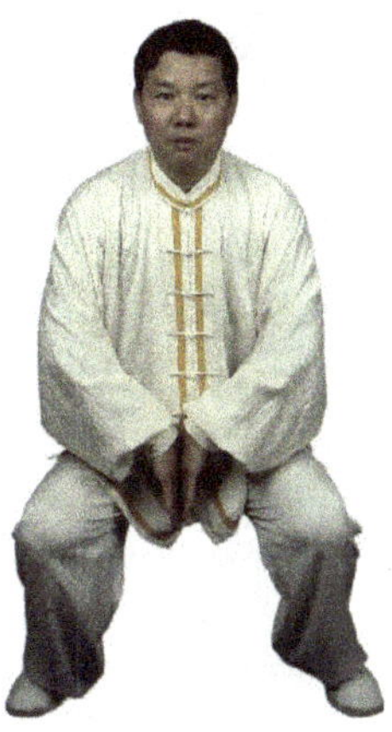

Illustration 11-7 Receive the Fruit, Collect Inside

The previous movement does not stop, the body's center of gravity sinks down, both legs bend at the knees to squat down changing to a horse stance. At the same time, both arms revolve inward, the shoulders relax and the elbows sink down, both palms from the front of the chest turn over and insert down, stopping below the abdomen in front of the lower Dan Tian, the fingertips point down, the backs of the hands stick to each other, the little finger side faces front. At the same time, the Dan Tian sticks outward, breathe out. The tongue rests on the lower palate, the teeth are slightly closed. The eyes look front; the intention is on circulating energy and breath down to the Dan Tian. (Illustration 11-7 and 11-8)

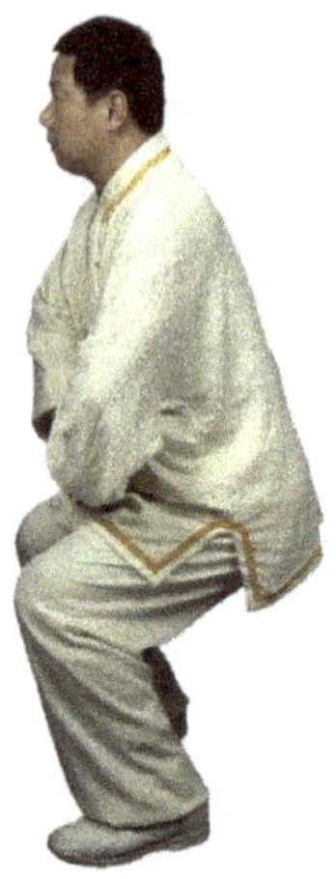

Illustration 11-8 Ape Washes its Face

5) Ape Washes its Face

These movement methods are entirely the same as for Both Appear Left posture, but the left and right sides are reversed (see Illustrations 11-1, 11-2, and 11-3)

6) Offering Fruit Right Posture

These movement methods are entirely the same as for Both Appear Left posture, but the left and right sides are reversed (see Illustration 11-4 and 11-5).

7) Turn the Body, Small Return

This movement method is entirely the same as for Pushing the Mountain Extremely Empty Initially (see Illustration 2-1). The previous movement does not stop, the next movement method is entirely the same as Extreme Emptiness Exercise, Blend the Elements with one breath (see Illustration 1-8).

Main Points and Functions

White Ape Presents Fruit Exercise uses bending and stretching to push down the inner breath and body fluid to return to the Dan Tian, the breath mainly circulates along the Dai Mai. The Dai Mai travels horizontally at the space between the waist and the abdomen, it connects the whole body vertically holding the meridians and channels restrained and pulled up, as if it were a belt. This has the effect of controlling the meridians, so they do not have random effects. The thoughts must focus on paying attention to three major points: The first major point is peacefulness, this means "everything bears yin and embraces yang, excited breath becomes peaceful," therefore, we must observe peace. The second major point is spirit, which means "A person's ears and eyes, how can they work for a long time and not rest, a person's energy and spirit, how can they leap and gallop and not be exhausted," therefore, it is important to guard it and not lose it. The third major point is breath, this refers to "the blood and breath are concentrated and sudden, without going beyond, then the chest and the belly will fill with breath and the intention will be focused," therefore work to guard the breath. When these three points are observed, the person will be peaceful, the spirit will be tranquil, and the inner breath will circulate.

When both hands hold the fruit in front of the body, the five fingers open around the outside to support, pushing forward, entering, they must go upward with an arc-shaped movement. In this way, gradually the effect will be to "set straight the body and expel evil." In setting straight the body and expelling evil, "setting straight" means correct inner breath, natural breath, and refers to the body's resistance to disease, to it's ability to maintain and protect good health; "evil" refers to irregular breath which has various detrimental factors. When people get sick, it means that the straight breath is not sufficient, the evil breath has invaded or the evil breath is too great. Earlier teachers said: "collect the straight breath inside", "disease is always looking for a place." Then "the straight and true" can enhance the upper body function of resistance.

Practice Method:

Each time, practice 6 times or 12 times to make one set, practicing again and again in succession is fine. The extent of the movement being larger or smaller, moving higher or lower is without restriction, depending on the age of the person practicing being older or younger, whether the physical strength is greater or lesser, and the weakness or strength in the body.

Acupuncture Points 点穴 (dian xue)

Lao Gong xue 劳宫穴 Palace of Toil PC-8[who]

Dai Mai 带脉 Girdling Vessel GIV, GB-26[who]

Zu Shao Yang Dan jing 足少阳胆经 Foot's Lesser Yang Gallbladder channel GB[who]

Cheng Jiang xue 承浆穴 Sauce Receptacle CV-24[who]

Yong Quan xue 涌泉穴 Bubbling Spring KC-1[who]

Shou Tai Yin Fei jing 手太阴肺经 Hand's Greater Yin Lung channel LU[who]

Jue Yin Xinbao jing 厥阴心包经 Reverting Yin Pericardium channel PC[who]

Yu Tang xue 玉堂穴 Jade Hall CV-18[who]

Xuan Guan qiao 玄关窍 Mysterious Gate opening (upper Dan Tian)

Set 12 Red Phoenix Faces the Sun Exercise

In Red phoenix faces the sun the breath flows to Heaven,
shoulders relax, elbows sink down, distinguish yin and yang.
From the breathing circulation methods and patterns,
one hundred years long life happy and healthy.

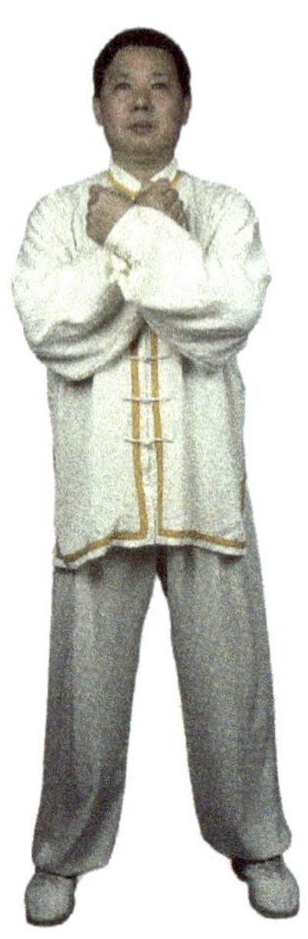

Illustration 12-1 Raise and Drill, Drop and Turn Over

1) Preparation

These movement methods are exactly the same as for Extreme Emptiness Exercise, Preparation Postures. (see Illustrations 1-1, 1-2, 1-3, 1-4)

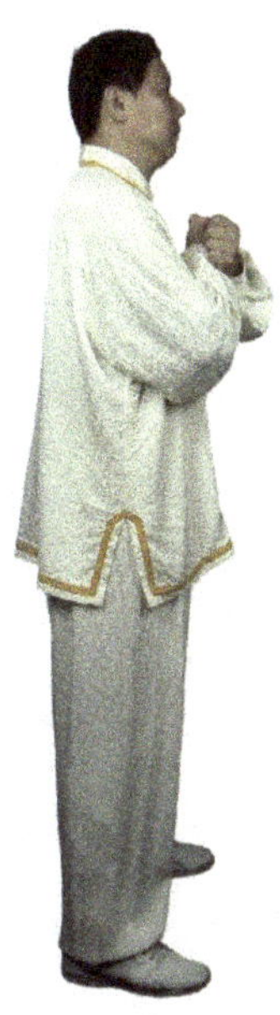

llustration 12-2 Raise and Drill, Drop and Turn Over

2) Raise, Drill, Drop, and Turn Over

The previous movement does not stop, both arms revolve outward, both palms change into fists and from the sides of the body rise to the front in an arc shape. The left fist on the outside; the right fist on the inside, crossed together, stopping in front of the chest. The backs of the fists face front, the centers of the fists face in, the heels of the palms Da Ling acupuncture points connect with the sides of the chest Zhou Rong acupuncture points. At the same time, the Dan Tian sinks inward, breathe in. The tongue rises against the upper palate, the teeth are lightly closed. The eyes are slightly closed, the intention is on the Bai Hui acupuncture point, the breath circulates through the foot Tai Yin Pi channel. (Illustration 12-1, 12-2)

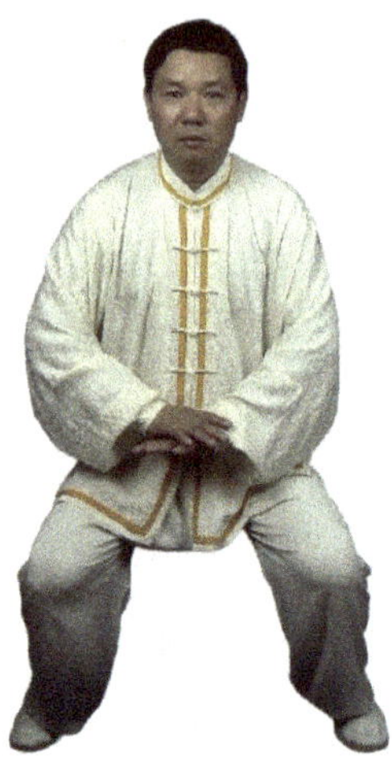

Illustration 12-3 Raise and Drill, Drop and Turn Over

The previous movement does not stop, the upper body center of gravity sinks down, both legs bend at the knees to squat down changing into a horse stance. At the same time, both arms revolve inward, both fists change into palms and press down in front of the abdomen (right above, left below). The fingertips slant towards the front, the palms face down. Also at the same time, the Dan Tian sticks outward, breathe out. The eyes look front and down, the intention is on raising the index finger. (Illustration 12-3)

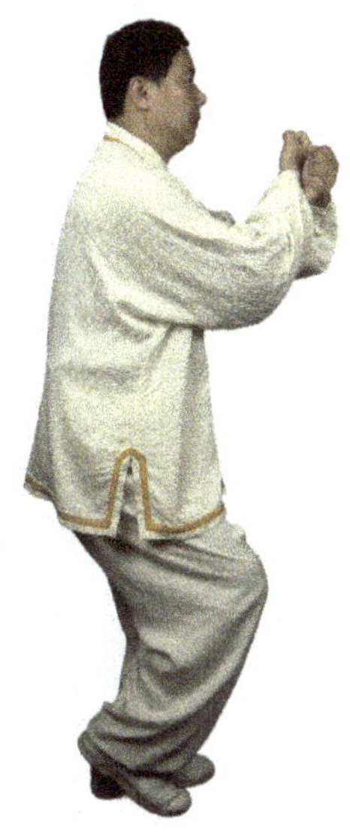

Illustration 12-4 Red Phoenix Left Posture

3) Red Phoenix Left Posture

The previous movement pauses slightly, the body's center of gravity shifts to the left leg, the body turns left 90 degrees, facing east. The right foot shifts to the outside of the left foot arch, the toes point to the ground changing to a right toe (ding bu) stance. At the same time, both arms revolve outward, the ten fingers bend changing to fists, from the front of the abdomen arc upward to the front, the right fist inside, the left outside, crossing and stopping in front of the chest. The right forearm's Nei Guan acupuncture point presses down from above the left lower arm Wai Guan acupuncture point, the backs of the fists face front, the palms face back. At the same time, the Dan Tian sinks inward, breathe in. The tongue rises against the upper palate, the teeth are lightly closed. The eyes follow the body's turning, the intention is on the Nei Guan and Wai Guan acupuncture points. (Illustration 12-4)

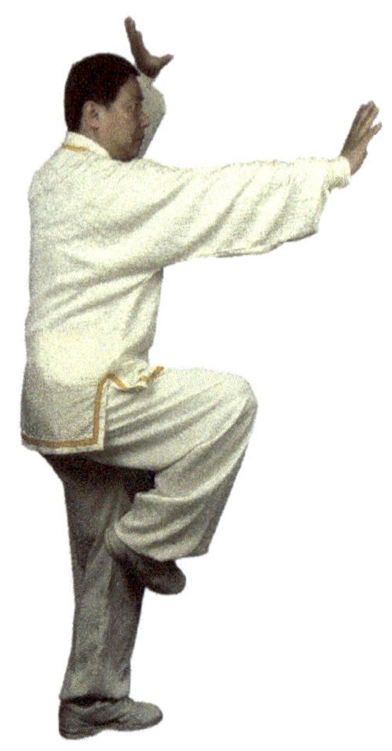

Illustration 12-5 Red Phoenix Left Posture

The previous movement does not stop, the left leg straightens to support, the right knee rises, the toes point down changing to a right single leg standing posture. At the same time as raising the leg, both arms revolve inward, the ten fingers extend open changing to palms. The left palm from the front of the chest rises upward in an arc shape with an arc at the bend of the elbow horizontally stopping above the crown of the head, the fingertips point right, the palm faces up; the right palm uses strength to slowly push out, the fingertips point up, the palm faces front. When pushing, the Dan Tian acupuncture point sticks outward, breathe out. The tongue rests on the lower palate, the teeth are slightly closed. The eyes look at the palm of the front hand, the intention is on both palms separating and pulling. (Illustration 12-5)

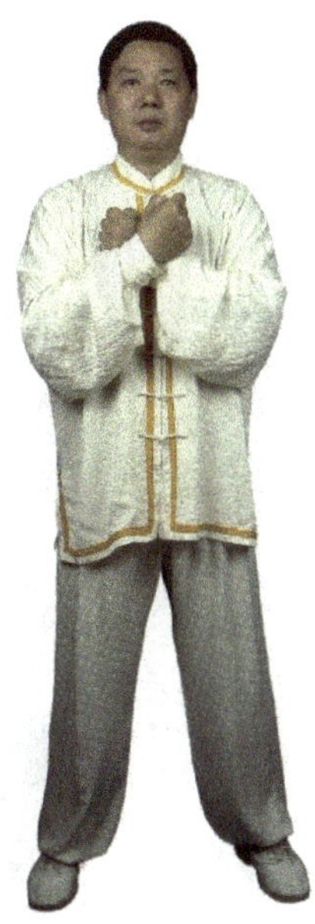

Illustration 12-6 Turn the Body, Connect the Breath

4) Turn the Body, Connect the Breath

The previous movement pauses slightly, the right foot to the back lowers to the ground, the body turns right 90 degrees, facing south. Both arms revolve outward, both palms change into fists and from the sides of the body rise to the front in an arc shape. The right fist is outside; the left fist inside, they form a cross and stop in front of the chest. The backs of the fists face front, the palms face in, the heels of the palm Da Ling acupuncture points press against the side of the chest Zhou Rong acupuncture points. Also at the same time, the Dan Tian sinks inward, breathe in. The tip of the tongue presses against the upper palate, the teeth are lightly closed. The eyes are slightly closed, the intention is at the Bai Hui acupuncture point, the breath circulates through the foot Da Yin Pi channel. (Illustration 12-6)

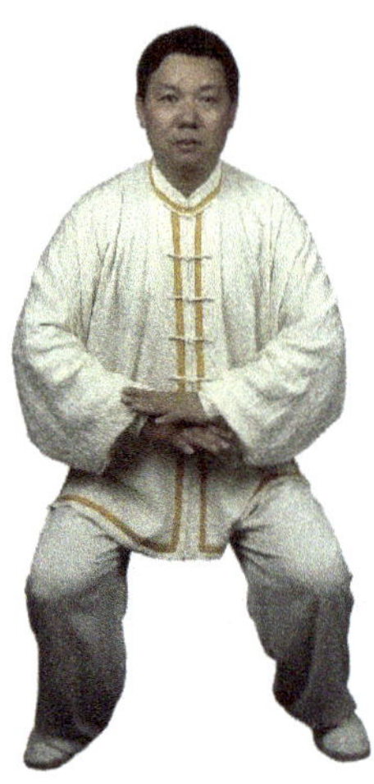

Illustration 12-7 Turn the Body, Connect the Breath

The previous movement does not stop, the upper body's center of gravity sinks down, both legs bend at the knees to squat down changing to a horse stance. At the same time, both arms revolve inward, both fists change into palms and press down in front of the abdomen (left on top, right on the bottom). The fingertips slant towards the front, the palms face down. At the same time, the Dan Tian sticks outward, breathe out. The eyes look front and down, the intention is on raising the index finger. (Illustration 12-7)

5) Red Phoenix Right Posture

These movement methods are entirely the same as for Red Phoenix Left posture, but the left and right sides are reversed (Illustration 12-4, 12-5)

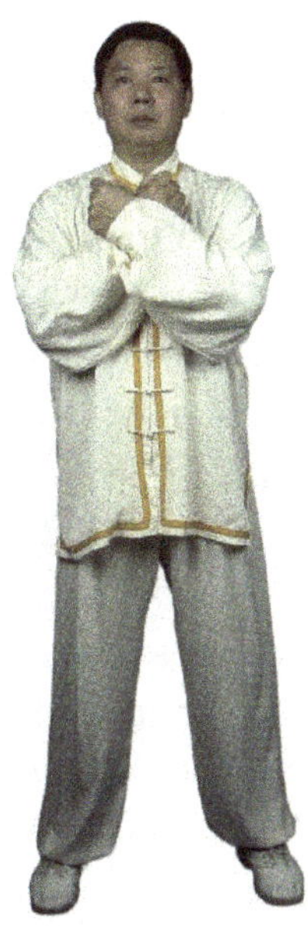

Illustration 12-8 Red Phoenix Right Posture

6) Return the Body to the Beginning Posture

The previous movement pauses slightly, the left foot lowers back to the ground, the body turns left 90 degrees, facing south, naturally standing straight. At the same time, both arms revolve outward, both palms change into fists again and return, the left fist on the outside and the right fist on the inside, crossing and stopping in front of the chest, the backs of the fist face front, the palms face inward. Also at the same time, the Dan Tian sinks inward, breathe in. The tongue rises against the upper palate, the teeth are slightly closed. The eyes follow the turning of the body, the intention is on the sides of the chest Zhou Rong acupuncture points. (Illustration 12-8)

This movement method is entirely the same as Extreme Emptiness Exercise, Blend the Elements with one breath (see Illustration 1-8).

Main Points and Functions:

Red Phoenix Flies to the Sun posture main purpose is "refine energy and transform inner breath", inner breath circulates through the large and small heavenly circles. When turning the body, use the waist to drive the movement of the whole body together, both hands are crossed at an angle and intersect in front of the chest, the palm center Lao Gong acupuncture point and the sides of the chest Zhou Rong acupuncture point face each other and attract each other. Raising the leg to stand on one leg and the rising posture, the forward palm pushing all must be harmonious and coordinated. The body must remain straight and stable, the whole body relaxed and the chest a little contained. When setting the foot, the fists and the center of gravity lowering are neat and consistent, maintaining it with constant practice. When practice has arrived at a certain level, then one can feel, when breathing out inner breath from the Dan Tian moves through the Hui Yin acupuncture point straight to the Yong Quan acupuncture point; when breathing in, the inner breath from the Yong Quan moves through the Hui Yin to arrive at the Ming Men, in this way it will naturally flow smoothly through the Chang Qiang acupuncture point. Next, the inner breath passes the Jia Ji acupuncture point and the Yu Zhen acupuncture point. The Jia Ji is located nine centimeters below the large vertebra, the Yu Zhen is at the back of the head below the Feng Fu acupuncture point.

When first practicing, the vertebra may feel like wood, then they may feel swollen, numb, warm, at last the inner breath from the Ming Men passes straight through the Jia Ji. When the Jia Ji outer breath feels it has reached about 6 centimeters wide, the Jia Ji can flow smoothly. Then, use this method to unblock the Yu Zhen xue, when the when the extension of breath feels six centimeters wide, the Yu Zhen acupuncture point can also flow.

On this basis, then the breath can be made to rise up to reach the Bai Hui acupuncture point, then it can feel like a warm wave flowing up, massaging the cerebellum, the top of the head feels cool and moist, the whole body incomparably comfortable.

After this, the breath descends, passing between both eyes, to the nose then traveling down to the Ren Zhong acupuncture point. At this time, bring the tongue down from the upper palate and rest it on the lower palate, slightly close the teeth, the breath then will travel down to the Cheng Jiang acupuncture point, connecting the both the Du Mai and Ren Mai, the inner breath from the Ren Mai returns down to the Dan Tian.

If when practicing, it happens that the tongue is parched, the mouth dry, the mind is upset, the thoughts are wasteful and there are signs of becoming angry, move the thoughts to the Yong Quan point, the Ming Men point, the Hui Yin point, to connect yin and yang together, join water and fire. After completing this step of workmanship, it is possible to prevent disease and dispel illness.

Practice Method:

Each time, practice 6 times or 12 times to make one set, practicing again and again in succession is fine. The extent of the movement being larger or smaller, moving higher or lower is without restriction, depending on the age of the person practicing being older or younger, whether the physical strength is greater or lesser, and the weakness or strength in the body.

Acupuncture Points 点穴 (dian xue)

Nei Guan 内关 Inner Pass PC-6[who]

Da Ling xue 大陵穴 Great Mound PC-7[who]

Zhou Rong xue 周荣穴 All-Round Flourishing SP-20[who]

Bai Hui xue 百会穴 Hundred Convergences GV-20[who]

Tai Yin Pi jing 太阴脾经 Greater Yin Spleen channel SP[who]

Wai Guan 外关 Outer Pass TB-5

Da Ling xue 大陵穴 Great Mound PC-7[who]

Zhou Rong xue 周荣穴 All-Round Flourishing SP-20[who]

Tai Yin Pi jing 太阴脾经 Greater Yin Spleen channel SP[who]

Lao Gong xue 劳宫穴 Palace of Toil PC-8[who]

Hui Yin 会阴 Meeting of Yin (perineum) CV-1[who]

Yong Quan xue 涌泉穴 Bubbling Spring KC-1[who]

Ming Men xue 命门穴 Life Gate GV-4[who]

Jia Ji xue 夹脊穴 Paravertebrals

Yu Zhen 玉枕 Jade Pillow BK-9[who]

Feng Fu xue 风府穴 Wind House GV-16[who]

Ren Zhong xue 人中穴 Human Center GV-26[who]

Cheng Jiang xue 承浆穴 Sauce Receptacle CV-24[who]

Ren Mai 任脉 Controlling Vessel; Conception Vessel CV[who]

Chang Qiang xue 长强穴 Long and Rigid GV-1[who]

Set 13 Stir the Grass to Seek the Snake Exercise

Hiding the flower in the armpit is not strange,

left sway, right close, so it is done.

Stir the grass to seek the snake right and left,

Intention and breath join to strengthen the foundation.

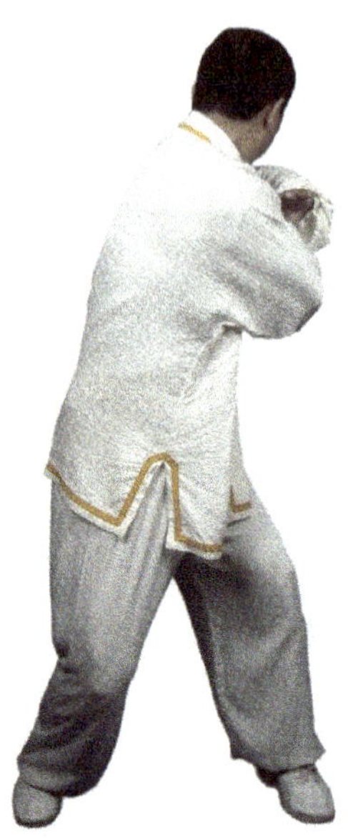

Illustration 13-1 Stirring the Grass to Seek the Snake Left

1) Preparation

These movement methods are exactly the same as for Extreme Emptiness Exercise, Preparation Postures. (see Illustrations 1-1, 1-2, 1-3, 1-4)

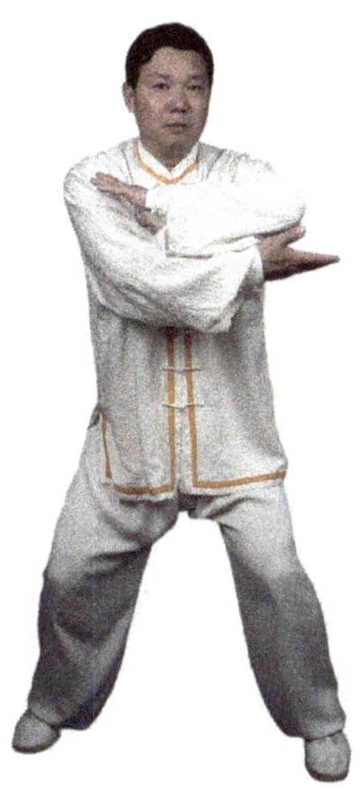

Illustration 13-2 Stirring the Grass to Seek the Snake Left

2) Stirring the Grass to Seek the Snake Left Posture

The previous movement pauses slightly, the right toes close inward, the body's center of gravity sinks between both legs changing to a bow horse stance. The right arm revolves outward, the right hand from the side of the body rises up and inserts to the left stopping under the left arm, the fingertips point left, the palm faces up, the palm center Lao Gong acupuncture point faces the underarm Ji Quan acupuncture point; the left hand rises to the right in an arc, stopping above the right elbow, the fingertips face right, the palm faces down. Also at the same time, the Dan tian sinks inward, breathe in. The tongue rises against the upper palate, the teeth are slightly closed. The eyes look toward the left front, the intention is on the breath passing through the Bai Hui acupuncture point. (Illustrations 13-1 and 13-2)

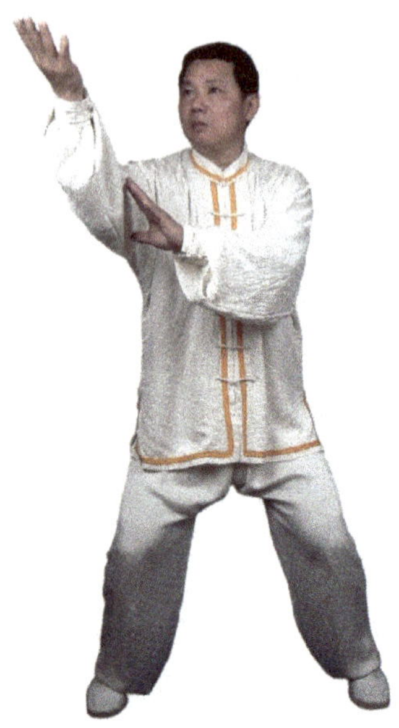

Illustration 13-3 Stirring the Grass to Seek the Snake Left

The previous movement does not stop, the body's center of gravity rises upward, the body turns right, both arms toward the right front and upward swing out. The right hand is above and slightly higher than the head; the left hand is below at the same height as the nose, stopping above the side of the right elbow joint. The fingertips of both hands point toward the front and up, the back of the hands face down. At the same time, the Dan tian sticks outward, breathe out. The tongue rests on the lower palate, the teeth are lightly closed. The eyes look at the right hand, the intention is on the lower arm Kong Zui acupuncture point, the breath and blood follow and circulate through the hand Tai Yin Fei channel. (Illustration 13-3)

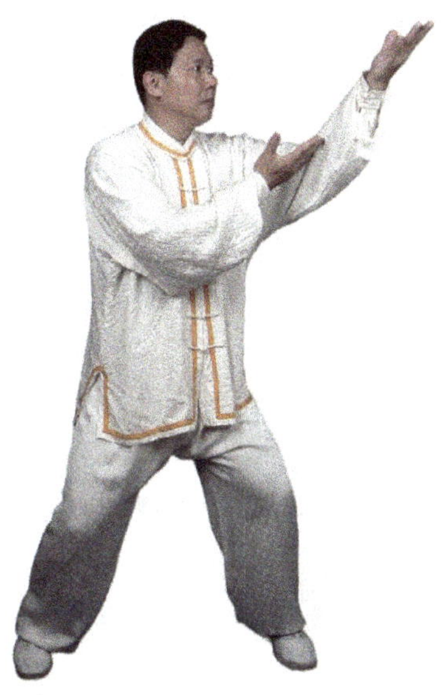

Illustration 13-4 Stirring the Grass to Seek the Snake Left

The previous movement pauses slightly, the body turns left, both arms revolve inward, the little finger side of the back of the hand and arm uses strength to turn over, both wrists cross changing to crossed hands, right below left above stopping at the left side of the head, the palms face inward and up, the fingertips point upward at an angle. Also at the same time, the Dan tian sinks inward, breathe in. The tongue rises against the upper palate, the teeth are slightly closed. The eyes follow the turning of the palms, the intention is on the wrist Shen Men acupuncture point. (Illustration 13-4)

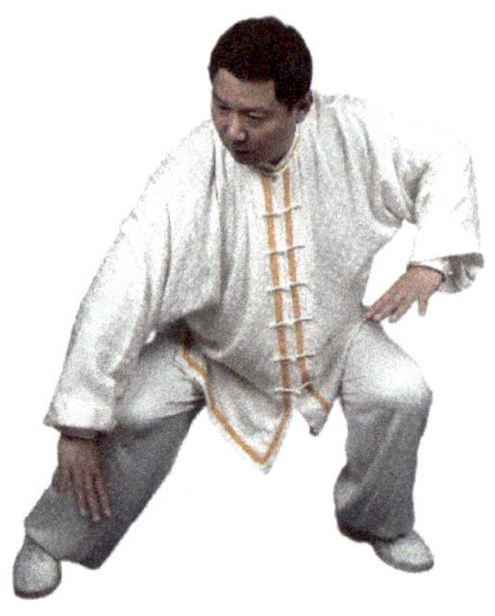

Illustration 13-5 Stirring the Grass to Seek the Snake Left

The previous movement does not stop, the body turns left. The body's center of gravity sinks down, the left leg bends at the knee to squat down, the right leg steps right half a step changing to right horizontal six four step. At the same time, both elbows open to the outside, both palms push down with strength, then separate to both sides, stopping below the knees. The palms face down, the little finger side faces front. Also at the same time, the Dan Tian sticks outward, breathe out. The tongue rests on the lower palate, the teeth are lightly closed. The eyes look toward the front and down, the intention is on both hands turning the grass to seek the snake, the inner breath and blood circulate through the hand's Yang Ming Da Chang channel. (Illustration 13-5)

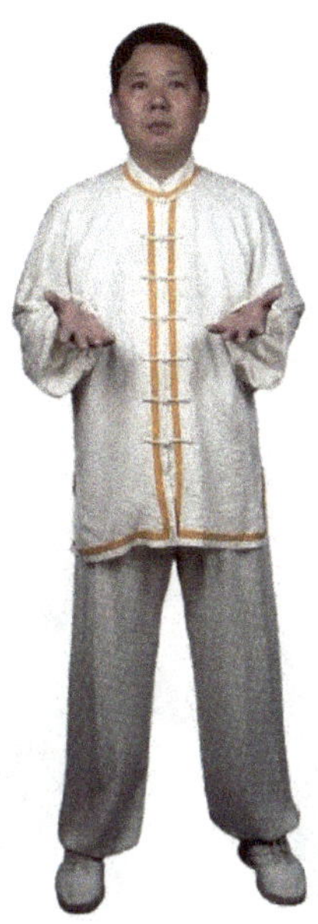

Illustration 13-6 Straighten the Body, Small Return

3) Straighten the Body, Small Return

The previous movement pauses slightly, the body turns to the right, facing south. After circulating the breath out and in two times, both legs extend to stand naturally. At the same time, both arms revolve to the outside; both hands together turn inward and rise upward, the heels of the palms stop just below both breasts. The fingertips of both hands point front, the palms face up. At the same time, the Dan Tian sinks inward, breathe in. The tongue rises against the upper palate, the teeth are slightly closed, the eyes look to the front. (Illustration 13-6)

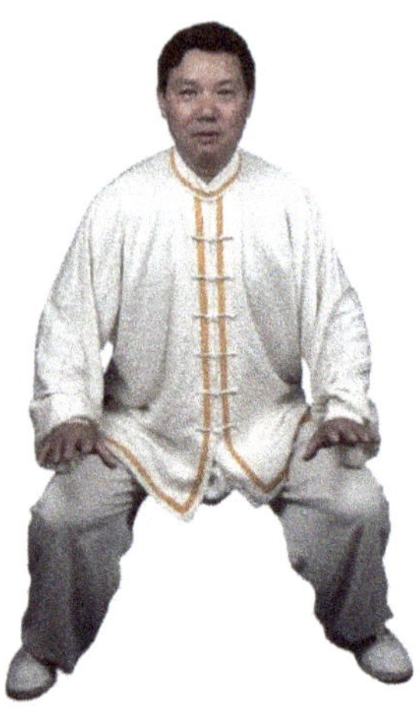

Illustration 13-7 Straighten the Body, Small Return

The previous movement does not stop, the body's center of gravity lowers, both legs bend at the knees to squat down changing to a horse stance. At the same time, both arms revolve inward and both elbows hold together, the hands turn toward the front of the body in an arc shape and press down, stopping in front of the abdomen. The palms face down, the fingertips point forward. At the same time, the Dan Tian sticks outward, breathe out. The tongue rests on the lower palate; the teeth are lightly closed. The eyes look slightly downward; the intention is at the Dan Tian, the breath circulates through both the Du Mai and the Ren Mai. (Illustration 13-7 and 13-8)

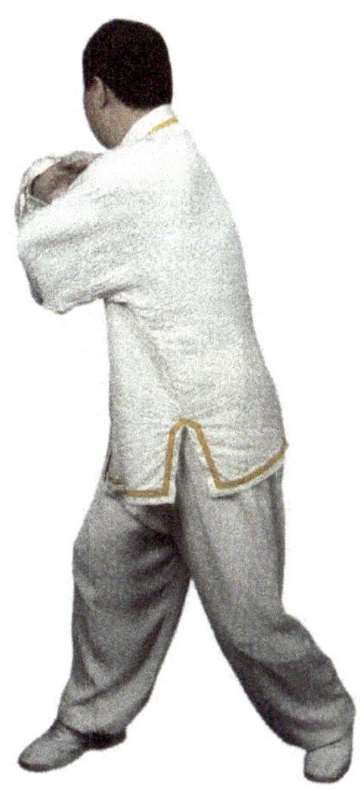

Illustration 13-8 Stirring the Grass to Seek the Snake Right

4) Stirring the Grass to Seek the Snake Right Posture

These movement methods are entirely the same as for Both Appear Left posture, but the left and right sides are reversed (see Illustrations 13-1, 13-2, 13-3, 13-4, 13-5)

5) Raise the Body, Return to the Beginning

This movement method is entirely the same as for Pushing the Mountain Extremely Empty Initially (see Illustration 2-1). The previous movement does not stop, the next movement method is entirely the same as Extreme Emptiness Exercise, Blend the Elements with one breath (see Illustration 1-8).

Main Points and Functions

In Stirring the Grass to Seek the Snake Exercise, the primary practice is to gather the spirit and strengthen the intention, in coiling down the foundation should be steady and firm. Strive to keep the hips relaxed and drawn back, the knees must be restrained and lively, the feet must be flat and steady, during the movement, the hands and feet must coordinate and move together. The hand accounts for three parts force, the foot uses seven parts strength, the five camps (organs) and the four extremities must join together as a whole, the breath circulates following the mind and intention, in Stirring the Grass to Seek the Snake nimble breath rises.

In gathering the spirit and strengthening the intention, then during practice there cannot be distracting thoughts. Once distracting thoughts arise, how can they be eliminated? Then, concentrate on one idea, use one idea to replace ten thousand ideas, and don't have don't want any thoughts. Certainly, at first the mind will be an ape and the intention a horse,[23] practice until the mind is calm and the spirit is peaceful, the spirit is at peace and the mind calm, the mind leading a wave to a calm state, this requires a complicated extensive change process.

If distracting thoughts emerge, then the hands will be busy and the feet confused, and become in a hurry the are forgotten and the feet become disorderly, then one becomes impatient, or the person simply does not practice, then in the whole lifetime, practice will still not be good. As everyone knows, the process of overcoming distracting thoughts, it is a progressive and profitable workmanship process. It is necessary to keep the thoughts focused during the exercise on the requirements for the channels and meridians, standing positions, and on the acupuncture points. As time goes by, the gathering the spirit and

---

[23] 心猿意马 (xin yuan yi ma) restless and whimsical

quieting the mind will be accomplished, using one thought to replace ten thousand thoughts and muddled thoughts.

Experts in the boxing arts and breath exercises all know, coiling downward cannot be loose or slack. If coiling downward is loose and slack, the whole body becomes empty, seeming like duckweed without roots. Practice to develop a deep and strong root. In practice only when the root is deep and the base solid, the circulation lively, only then will the effects be felt everywhere.

During the exercise, it is required that everything be loose, quiet, round, and lively, all come from and out of the root. If this principle can be firmly grasped, naturally and smoothly changing the condition can be achieved.

Practice Method

Each time, practice 6 times or 12 times to make one set, practicing again and again in succession is fine. The extent of the movement being larger or smaller, moving higher or lower is without restriction, depending on the age of the person practicing being older or younger, whether the physical strength is greater or lesser, and the weakness or strength in the body.

Acupuncture Points 点穴 (dian xue)

Lao Gong xue 劳宫穴 Palace of Toil PC-8[who]

Ji Quan xue 极泉穴 Highest Spring HT-1[who]

Bai Hui xue 百会穴 Hundred Convergences GV-20[who]

Kong Zui 孔最 Collection Hole LU-6[who]

Shou Tai Yin Fei jing 手太阴肺经 Hand's Greater Yin Lung Channel LU[who]

Shen Men xue 神门穴 Spirit Gate HT-7[who]

Shou Yang Ming Dachang Jing 手阳明大肠经 Hand's Yang Brightness Large Intestine channel LI[who]

Du Mai 督脉 Governing Vessel GV[who]

Ren Mai 任脉 Controlling Vessel; Conception Vessel CV[who]

Set 14 Dragon and Tiger Join Together Exercise

West mountain white tiger is unrestrained,

Eastern green dragon is unstoppable.

Dragon and tiger join together, metal and wood combine;

desire is subdued and becomes a golden pill.

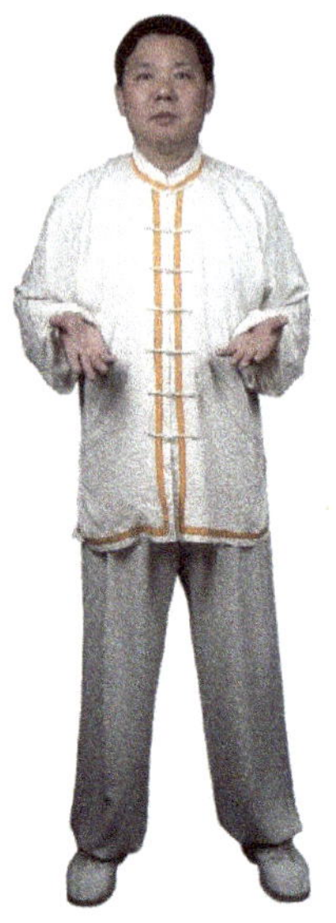

Illustration 14-1 Metal and Wood Combine Together

1) Preparation

These movement methods are exactly the same as for Extreme Emptiness Exercise, Preparation Postures. (see Illustrations 1-1, 1-2, 1-3, 1-4)

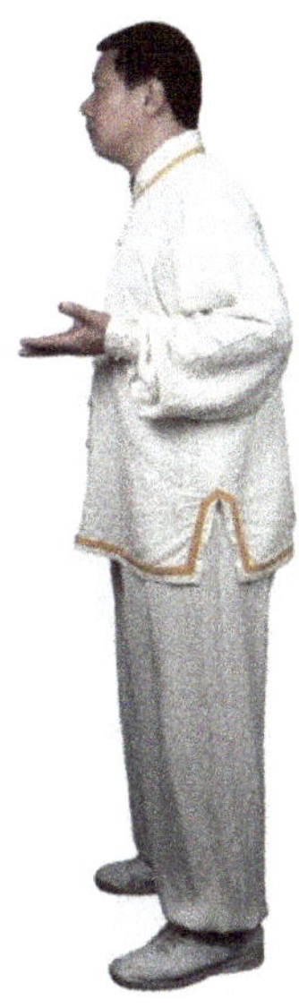

Illustration 14-2 Metal and Wood Combine Together

2) Metal and Wood Combine Together

The previous movement pauses slightly. After circulating the breath out and in two times, both legs extend to stand naturally. At the same time, both arms revolve to the outside; both hands together turn inward and rise upward, the heels of the palms stop just below both breasts. The fingertips of both hands point front, the palms face up. At the same time, the Dan Tian sinks inward, breathe in. The tongue rises against the upper palate, the teeth are slightly closed, the eyes look to the front. (Illustrations 14-1 and 14-2)

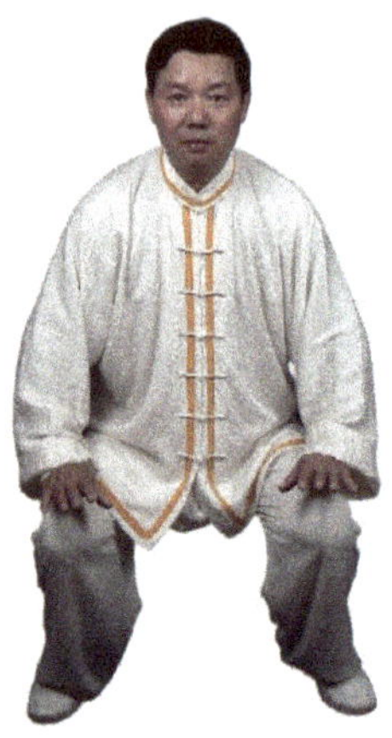

Illustration 14-3 Metal and Wood Combine Together

The previous movement does not stop, the body's center of gravity lowers, both legs bend at the knees to squat down changing to a horse stance. At the same time, both arms revolve inward and both elbows hold together, the hands turn toward the front of the body in an arc shape and press down, stopping in front of the abdomen. The palms face down, the fingertips point forward. At the same time, the Dan Tian sticks outward, breathe out. The tongue rests on the lower palate; the teeth are lightly closed. The eyes look slightly downward; the intention is at the Dan Tian, the breath circulates through both the Du Mai and the Ren Mai. (Illustration 14-3)

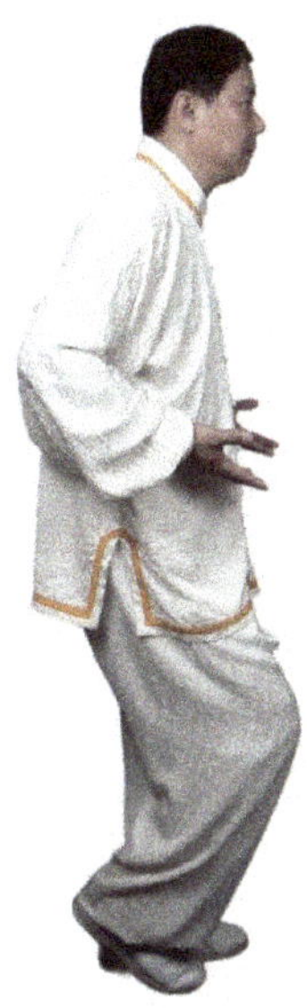

Illustration 14-4 Dragon and Tiger Join Together Left Posture

3) Dragon and Tiger Join Together Left Posture

The previous movement pauses slightly, the body turns left 90 degrees, the left leg bends at the knee to squat, the right foot pulls in near the heel, stopping at the inside of left foot, the toes point to the ground, the body's center of gravity sinks onto the left foot, changing to a right set stance.[24] At the same time, both palms from below the navel rise up to the left front in an arc shape, stopping in front of the chest at the Zhong Ting acupuncture points. The middle fingers of both hands connect, the fingertips point front and down, the palms face inward and up. At the same time, the Dan Tian sinks inward, breathe in. The tip of the tongue presses against the upper palate, the teeth are slightly closed. The eyes follow the motion of the body, the intention is on the index finger Shang Yang acupuncture point, the breath circulates through the hand Yang Ming Da Chang channel. (Illustration 14-4)

[24] Ding bu 丁步 is a standard stepping method in many martial arts.

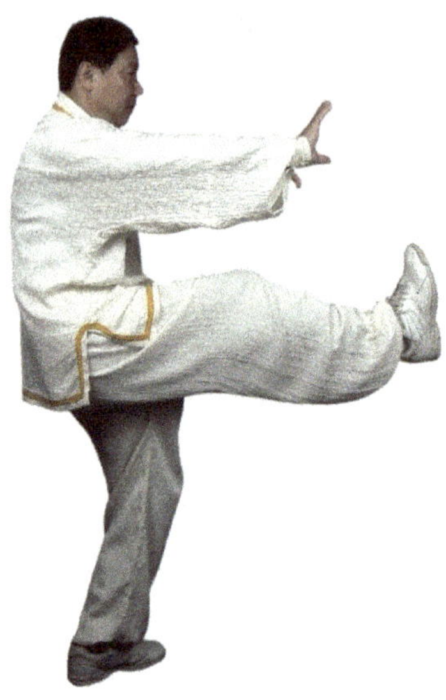

Illustration 14-5 Dragon and Tiger Join Together Left Posture

The previous movement does not stop, the left leg is solid and the knee is straight; the right knee bends and rises, the sole of the foot uses strength to extend out, at the same height as the hip, the toes point up, the center of the foot faces front. At the same time, both arms revolve inward, using the shoulders to promote the elbows, use the elbows to set the wrists, shoulders, elbows, wrists these three joints use strength to cause the palms to push outward, at the same height as the shoulders. The fingertips face each other, the palms face front. At the same time, the Dan Tian sticks outward, breathe out. The tongue rests on the lower palate, the teeth are lightly closed. The eyes look through the space between the fingers of the hands, the intention is on joining the mind and the kidneys. (Illustration 14-5)

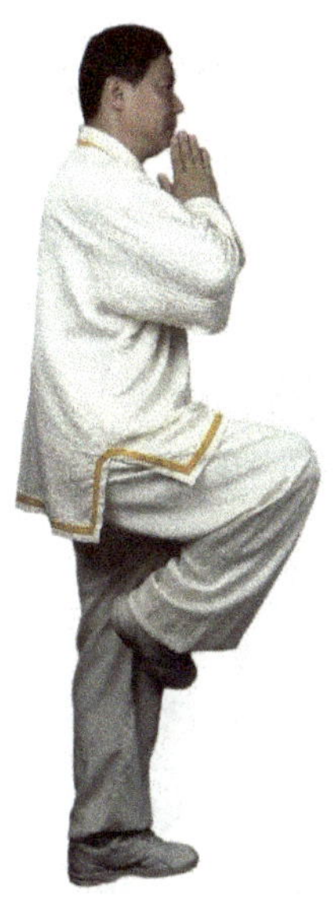

Illustration 14-6 Golden Pheasant Stands on One Leg

4) Golden Pheasant Stands on One Leg

The previous movement pauses slightly, the left leg extends straight and supports the body; the right leg is bent at the knee with the toes pulled back and pointed down, the front of the foot stretches straight changing to a right single leg standing posture. At the same time, both arms slightly revolve toward the outside, the heels of both palms draw close, the thumb tips stop below the lip at the Cheng Jiang acupuncture point. The fingertips face up, the little finger side faces front. Also at the same time, the Dan Tian sinks inward, breathe in. The tongue rises against the upper palate, the teeth are slightly closed. The eyes look toward the front and down. The intention is on the upper lip Ren Zhong acupuncture point, the breath rises along the Du Mai upward to the crown of the head. (Illustration 14-6)

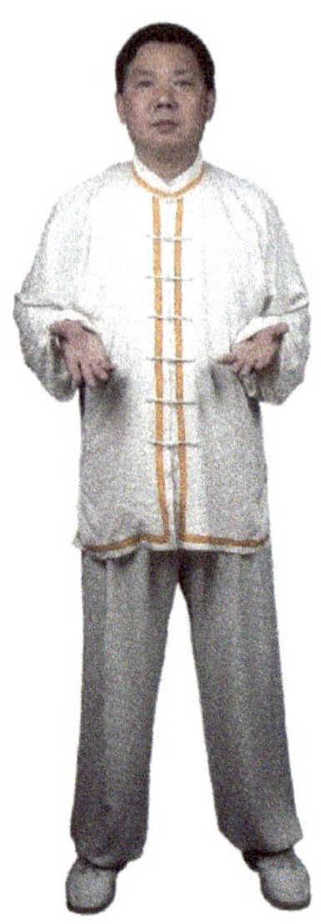

Illustration 14-7 Golden Pheasant Stands on One Leg

The previous movement does not stop, the body turns right 90 degrees. The right leg lowers to the ground, the left toes close inward, facing south and naturally standing straight. This movement method is completely the same as Extreme Emptiness Exercise, Blend the Elements with One Breath. (Illustration 14-7)

5) Dragon and Tiger Join Together Right Posture

These movement methods are entirely the same as for Dragon and Tiger Join Together Left posture, but the left and right sides are reversed (see Illustrations 14-1, 13-2, 13-3, 13-4, 13-5)

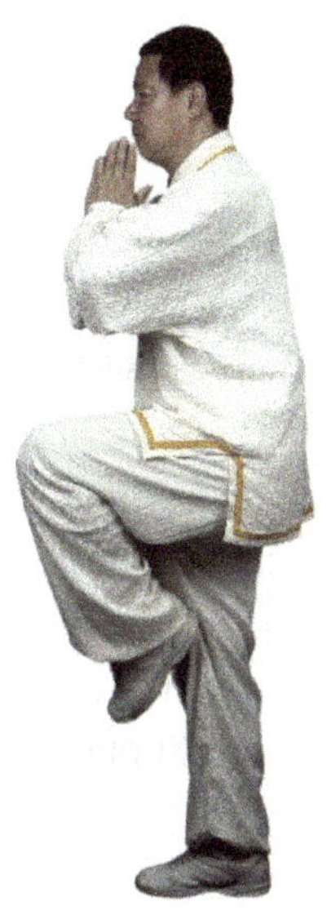

Illustration 14-8 Stand on One Leg Returning Posture

6) Stand on One Leg Returning Posture

The previous movement pauses slightly, the right leg extends straight and supports the body, the left leg is bent at the knee with the toes pulled back and pointed down, the front of the foot stretches straight changing into a left single leg standing posture. At the same time, both arms slightly revolve toward the outside, the heels of both palms draw close, the index fingers stop below the nose at the Ren Zhong acupuncture point, the fingertips face up, the little finger side faces front. At the same time, the Dan Tian sinks inward, breathe in. The tip of the tongue presses against the upper palate, the teeth are slightly closed. The eyes slightly look down, the intention is on the Ren Zhong acupuncture point, the breath rises through the Du Mai upward to the crown of the head. (Illustration 14-8)

This movement method is entirely the same as Extreme Emptiness Exercise, Blend the Elements with one breath (see Illustration 1-8).

Main Points and Functions:

During the practice of Dragon and Tiger Join Together Exercise, one must always strive to connect the mind with the intention, connect the intention with the breath, connect the breath with the force (movement). In other words, when one limb moves, one hundred limbs move simultaneously. Quiet as a mountain standing majestic and upright, moving as fast as thunder, one cannot cover the ears. Use the mind and spirit to gather and circulate the thoughts, observing the acupuncture points, various places, use the thoughts to gather and circulate the inner breath, following along the tiny heavenly circle, the small heavenly circle, and the large heavenly circle; the internal breath circulation and the movements in the exercises must be connected and coordinated, force cannot be separated from the intention, the intention and the inner breath must be connected. The Dan Tian sinks inward, raise the kidney water up to the brain, strike forward and down, the Mysterious Gate opening connects with the heart, then the heart fire and the kidney water join together, then travel down to the Dan Tian, the Dan Tian is full and the body is strong as stone. "Tiger" is a metaphor for primal energy, primal energy is created within kidney breath. The kidneys belong to Kan Gua,[25] which belongs to water. So it is said "the tiger is born beside water." "Dragon" is a metaphor for primal spirit, primal spirit is created in the fluid of the heart. The heart belongs to Li Gua,[26] which belongs to fire. So it is said "the dragon rises from within fire."

---

[25] 坎卦 (Kan Gua) the Abysmal; from the ba gua (eight trigrams)

[26] 离卦 (Li Gua) the Clinging; from the ba gua (eight trigrams)

It is also said that human nature belongs to wood, wood stands in the East, with the Zhen trigram, in the human body it belongs to the liver, and therefore it is called the Green Dragon; energy is human passion, which belongs to gold, gold stands in the West, with the Dui trigram, in the human body it belongs to the lungs, so it is also called the White Tiger.

Using the five elements destruction theory, metal can destroy wood, therefore, passion often damages the nature. During practice of Dragon and Tiger Join Together, one must sincerely intend to restrain, to subdue the dragon and restrict the tiger, to make them join into one. Between metal and wood there is no space, the nature and the energy submit and are refined to become the Golden Elixir.

Through concentrated thoughts, the mind becomes quiet, the body relaxed, to achieve restoring the mind and spirit, the mind and breath then can play a role in governing the functions of blood movement.

After practicing this method, the essential breath will be recharged, not only can "original yin, original yang" mutually aid and support, and also the kidney water can also connect with the heart fire, if the heart and kidney are not joined then heart palpitations, insomnia, nocturnal emissions, and other symptoms may appear and can be improved. In addition, the functions that coordinate the heart and internal organs[27] can be strengthened.

---

[27] 脏腑 (zang fu) the internal organs including, heart liver spleen, lungs, kidneys, stomach, gall bladder, intestines, and bladder

Practice Method

Each time, practice 6 times or 12 times to make one set, practicing again and again in succession is fine. The extent of the movement being larger or smaller, moving higher or lower is without restriction, depending on the age of the person practicing being older or younger, whether the physical strength is greater or lesser, and the weakness or strength in the body.

Acupuncture Points 点穴 (dian xue)

Du Mai 督脉 Governing Vessel GV[who]

Ren Mai 任脉 Controlling Vessel; Conception Vessel CV[who]

Zhong Ting xue 中庭穴 Center Palace CV-16[who]

Shang Yang xue 商阳穴 Shang Yang LI-1[who]

Shou Yang Ming Dachang jing 手阳明大肠经 Hand's Yang Brightness Large Intestine channel LI[who]

Cheng Jiang xue 承浆穴 Sauce Receptacle CV-24[who]

Ren Zhong xue 人中穴 Human Center GV-26[who]

Xuan Guan qiao 玄关窍 Mysterious Gate opening (upper Dan Tian)

Set 15 Coiling Snake Exercise

Coiling snake folds spinning into one root,
from the nose, regular fine breathing
seems continuous and unbroken.
Refine and change hundred treasures
according to the intention in the Dan,
so energy transforms breath and breath supports life.

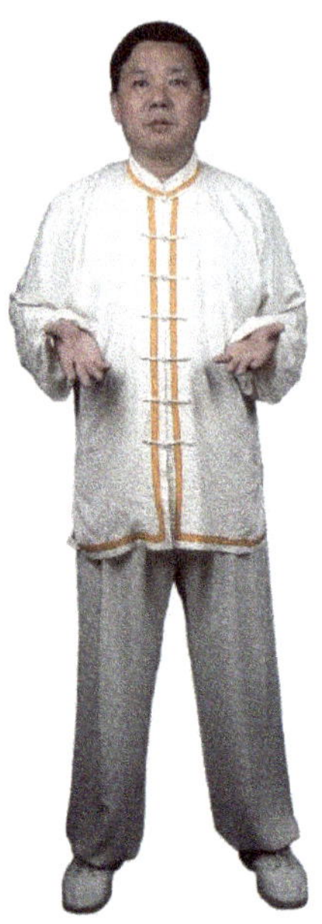

Illustration 15-1 Above and Below Connect the Breath

1) Preparation

These movement methods are exactly the same as for Extreme Emptiness Exercise, Preparation Postures. (see Illustrations 1-1, 1-2, 1-3, 1-4)

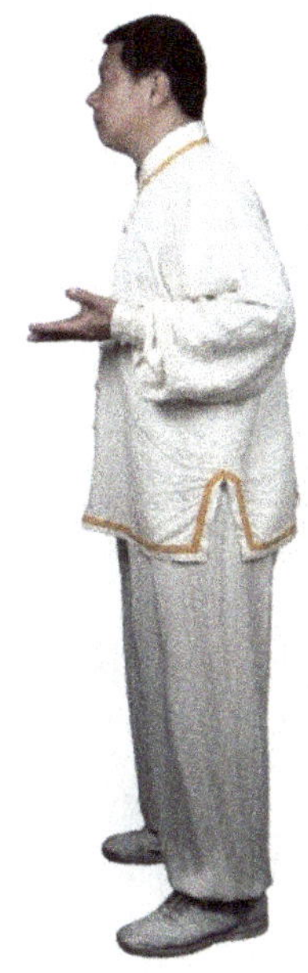

Illustration 15-2 Above and Below Connect the Breath

2) Above and Below Connect the Breath

The previous movement pauses slightly. After circulating the breath out and in two times, both legs extend to stand naturally. At the same time, both arms revolve to the outside; both hands together turn inward and rise upward, the heels of the palms stop just below both breasts. The fingertips of both hands point front, the palms face up. At the same time, the Dan Tian sinks inward, breathe in. The tongue rises against the upper palate, the teeth are slightly closed, the eyes look to the front. (Illustration 15-1 and 15-2)

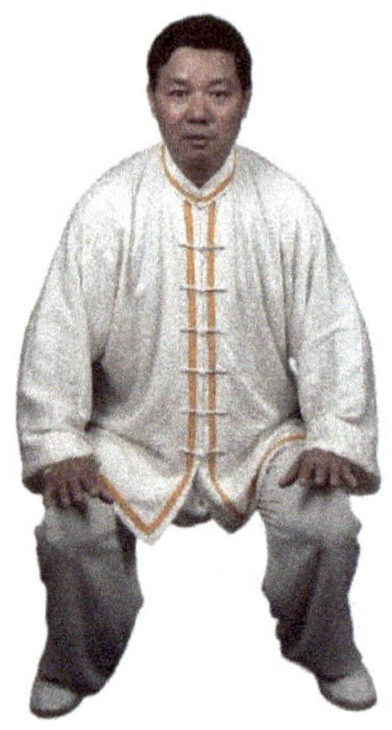

Illustration 15-3 Above and Below Connect the Breath

The previous movement does not stop, the body's center of gravity lowers, both legs bend at the knees to squat down changing to a horse stance. At the same time, both arms revolve inward and both elbows hold together, the hands turn toward the front of the body in an arc shape and press down, stopping in front of the abdomen. The palms face down, the fingertips point forward. At the same time, the Dan Tian sticks outward, breathe out. The tongue rests on the lower palate; the teeth are lightly closed. The eyes look slightly downward; the intention is at the Dan Tian, the breath circulates through both the Du Mai and the Ren Mai. (Illustration 15-3)

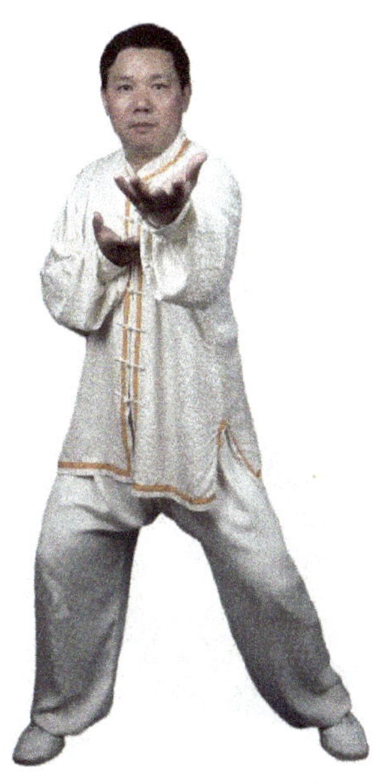

Illustration 15-4 Coiling Snake Left Posture

3) Coiling Snake Left Posture

The previous movement pauses slightly, the body turns slightly to the left, the body's center of gravity rises upward, facing south and naturally standing straight, erect, raise the heel. Both arms revolve outward, both hands from below the navel rise and press up to the left front in an arc shape. The left palm is in front and above, at the same height as the shoulders, the palm faces up, the fingertips point front; the right palm fingertips point at an angle to the inside of the left elbow joint, the palm faces up. Also at the same time, the Dan Tian sinks inward, breathe in. The tongue rises against the upper palate, the teeth are slightly closed. The eyes follow the left palm movement, the intention is on lifting the Yong Quan acupuncture point upward. (Illustration 15-4)

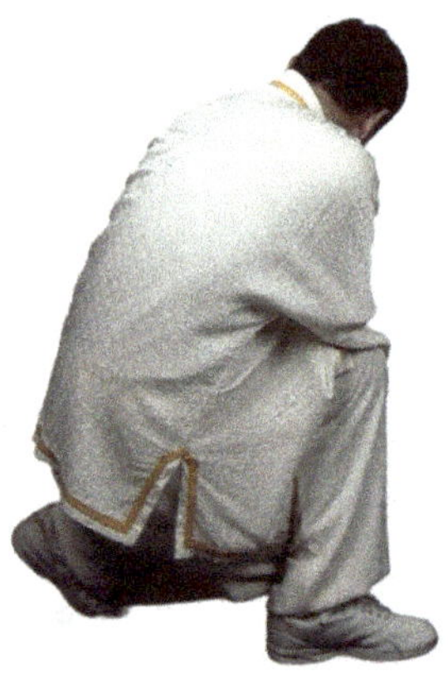

Illustration 15-5 Coiling Snake Left Posture

The previous movement does not stop, the body turns left, both legs cross and squat down at the same time, the whole left foot remains on the ground and opens outward, the heel of the right foot leaves the ground, the center of gravity shifts to the left leg changing to a left coiling snake stance. At the same time, both arms revolve inward, the left palm returns to a position in front of the chest, the fingertips point up, the palm faces right; the right palm inserts downward above the right heel, the fingers point at an angle to the right heel, the palm faces the right calf. At the same time, the Dan Tian sticks outward, breathe out. The tongue rests on the lower palate, the teeth are lightly closed. The eyes follow the body motion, the intention is on the Shen Shu acupuncture point, the breath circulates through the foot Tai Yang Pang Guang channel. (Illustration 15-5)

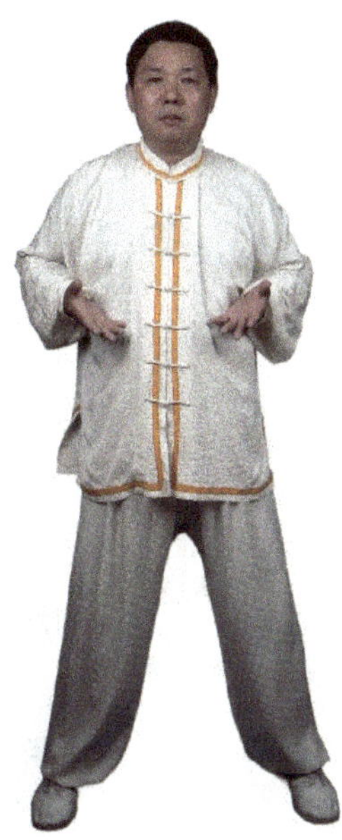

Illustration 15-6 Turn Right, Small Return

4) Turn Right, Small Return

The previous movement pauses slightly, after circulating the breath in and out two times, the body's center of gravity rises, the body turns toward the right, still facing south. At the same time, both arms revolve to the outside; both hands together turn inward and rise upward, the heels of the palms stop just below both breasts. The fingertips of both hands point front, the palms face up. At the same time, the Dan Tian sinks inward, breathe in. The tongue rises against the upper palate, the teeth are slightly closed, the eyes look to the front. (Illustration 15-6)

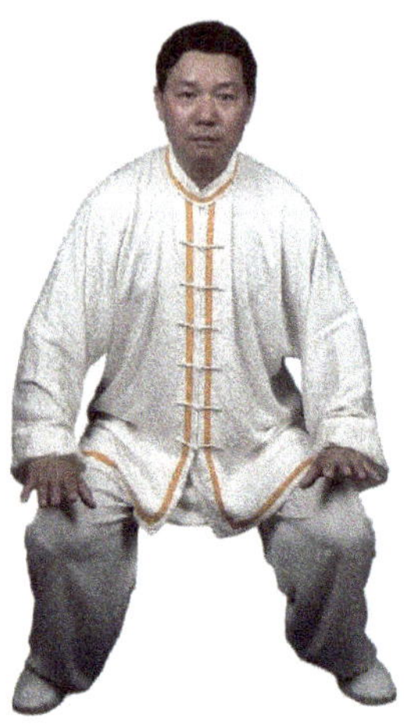

Illustration 15-7 Turn Right, Small Return

The previous movement does not stop, the body's center of gravity lowers, both legs bend at the knees to squat down changing to a horse stance. At the same time, both arms revolve inward and both elbows hold together, the hands turn toward the front of the body in an arc shape and press down, stopping in front of the abdomen. The palms face down, the fingertips point forward. At the same time, the Dan Tian sticks outward, breathe out. The tongue rests on the lower palate; the teeth are lightly closed. The eyes look slightly downward; the intention is at the Dan Tian, the breath circulates through both the Du Mai and the Ren Mai. (Illustration 15-7, 15-8)

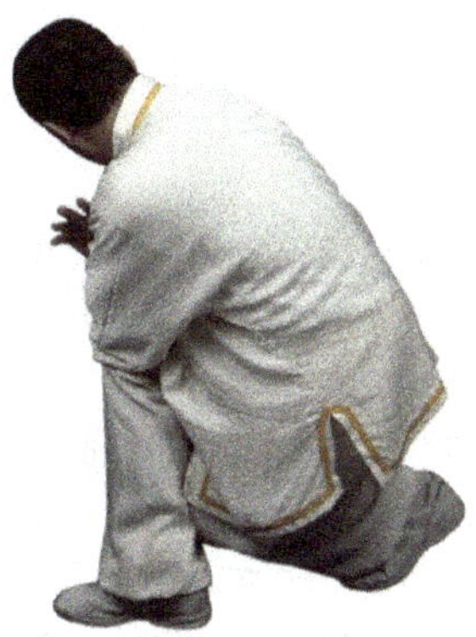

Illustration 15-8 Coiling Snake Right Posture

5) Coiling Snake Right Posture

These movement methods are entirely the same as for Coiling Snake Left posture, but the left and right sides are reversed (see Illustrations 15-4, 15-5).

6) Transform the Breath, Cultivate the Body

This movement method is entirely the same as for Pushing the Mountain Extremely Empty Initially (see Illustration 2-1). The previous movement does not stop, the next movement method is entirely the same as Extreme Emptiness Exercise, Blend the Elements with one breath (see Illustration 1-8).

Main Points and Functions:

In practicing Coiling Snake Exercise, the palm inserts downward with force, it must be joined together with the other hand rising and piercing strength. Both arms must hold close, the hips must be relaxed, the anus must lift, the shoulders must be closed, the elbows must sink, the head must be lifted. Use the waist to drive the turning movement of the whole body, and with the movement of both legs bending at the knees, crossing and squatting down together, coordinated, neat and consistent.

Coiling Snake Exercise is primarily to develop waist flexibility and circulate the inner breath through the large heavenly circle. The waist and spine during the whole movement play a dominant role, and must remain straight. Due to the demands of the action, the movement may contract, sway, bend down to help the internal breath circulate. The whole body rises and lowers, very much like a twisting rope, in the speed of the movements there is a kind of resilient strength. Sway the arms and hold the hips, the whole body rolls. The inner breath circulates through the large heavenly circle, this is Wudang Qigong's process of "practicing breath and transforming the spirit." It is through practicing the foundations of the small heavenly circle raising, through the study and practice of circulating the internal breath, that the spirit is made to connect with the breath, closely connected with the vigor and strength, combined as one and inseparable. Inner breath circulation routes, except the Du Mai, Ren Mai, small heavenly circle, can be included in the flow through other channels and meridians.

In practicing Wudang Qigong, one can't at once be an expert or be stubborn. The external form must smoothly, naturally, invisibly increase in strength. Inside the whole body connects with the Yuan Guan, invisibly increasing nimble breath. The thought must seek to be calm and natural, the intention and breath flow together, refining and combining, inhale softly, exhale slightly. Ultimately, the breathing, the thoughts, the sprint and breath are combined and naturally together joined.

Practice Method

Each time, practice 6 times or 12 times to make one set, practicing again and again in succession is fine. The extent of the movement being larger or smaller, moving higher or lower is without restriction, depending on the age of the person practicing being older or younger, whether the physical strength is greater or lesser, and the weakness or strength in the body.

Acupuncture Points 点穴 (dian xue)

Du Mai 督脉 Governing Vessel GV[who]

Ren Mai 任脉 Controlling Vessel; Conception Vessel CV[who]

Yong Quan xue 涌泉穴 Bubbling Spring KC-1[who]

Shen Shu xue 肾俞穴 Kidney BL-23[who]

Zu Tai Yang Pang Guang jing 足太阳膀胱经 Foot's Greater Yang Bladder channel BL[who]

Set 16 White Snake Sticks out its Tongue Exercise

In White Snake Sticks out its Tongue observe the breath inside,
using skill and using intent swing and sway the head.
Surging rivers return to the ocean,
use stillness and wait for the movement,
excellent and unhurried.

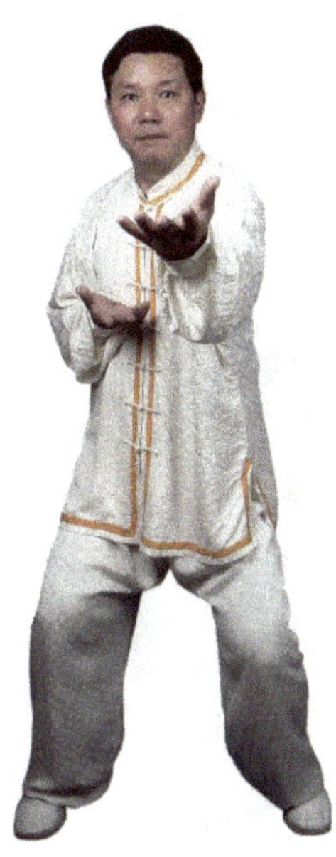

Illustration 16-1 White Snake Sticks out its Tongue Left Posture

1) Preparation

These movement methods are exactly the same as for Extreme Emptiness Exercise, Preparation Postures. (see Illustrations 1-1, 1-2, 1-3, 1-4)

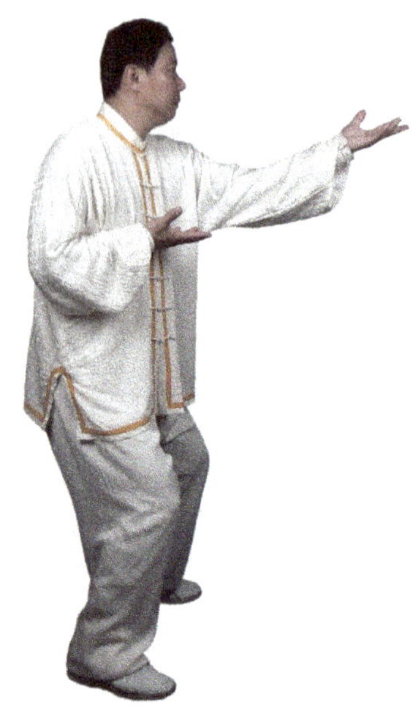

Illustration 16-2 White Snake Sticks out its Tongue Left Posture

2) White Snake Sticks out its Tongue Left Posture

The previous movement pauses slightly, the body slightly turns left, both arms revolve outward, the palms from the sides of the body forward to the left rise and press up in an arc shape The left palm is in front of and at the same height as the nose, the palm faces up, the fingertips point front; the right palm stops in front of the left shoulder, the fingertips point front, the palm faces up. At the same time, the Dan Tian sinks inward, breathe in. The tongue rises against the upper palate, the teeth are slightly closed. The eyes look at the left palm, the intention is on the hand center Lao Gong acupuncture point, the crown of the head center Bai Hui acupuncture point, and the foot center Yong Quan., the three centers inhale upper, middle and lower breath. (Illustrations 16-1 and 16--2)

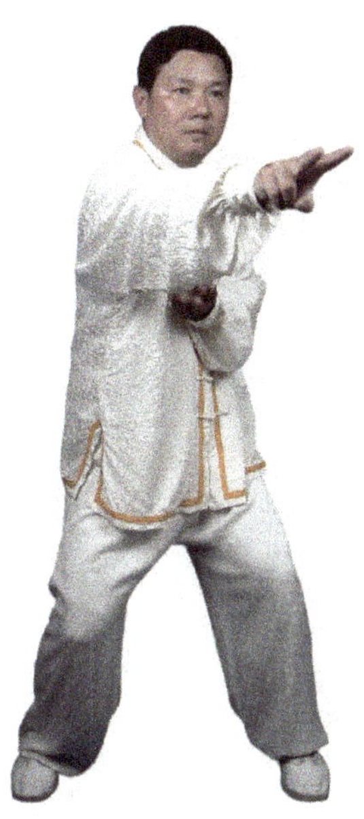

Illustration 16-3 White Snake Sticks out its Tongue Left Posture

The previous movement does not stop, the body slightly turns toward the right, the body's center of gravity sinks down, both legs bend at the knees to squat down changing to a horse stance. At the same time, both palms' index finger and middle finger extend straight and separate, the remaining three fingers bend to the center of the hand, the thumb presses on the ring finger and little finger above the first of the finger joints. The right palm from the right side of the chest rises to the front turning over and poking out, at the same height as the nose, the fingertips point front, the palm faces down; the left palm coordinates but the movement is inward and backward, stopping below the left breast, the fingertips point forward, the palm faces up. Also at the same time, the Dan Tian sticks outward, gradually breathe out. The tongue rests on the lower palate, the teeth are lightly closed. The eyes look at the fingers of the right hand, the intention is on twisting the waist and pulling with the palm. (Illustration 16-3)

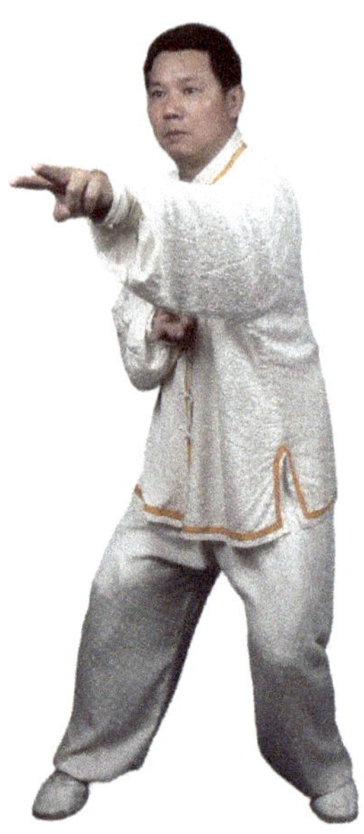

Illustration 16-4 White Snake Sticks out its Tongue Left Posture

The previous movement does not stop, the body slightly turns right, both hands' finger positions do not change. The left arm rises up and extends forward, the left palm from the left side of the chest stabs out forward, at the same height as the nose, the fingertips point front, the palm faces down; the right arm presses down; the right palm coordinates turning and returning, stopping below the right breast, fingertips pointing front, the palm facing up. Also at the same time, the Dan Tian continues turning outward, gradually breathe out. The tongue rests on the lower palate, the teeth are lightly closed. The eyes look at the fingers of the left palm, the intention is on the Dan Tian. (Illustration 16-4)

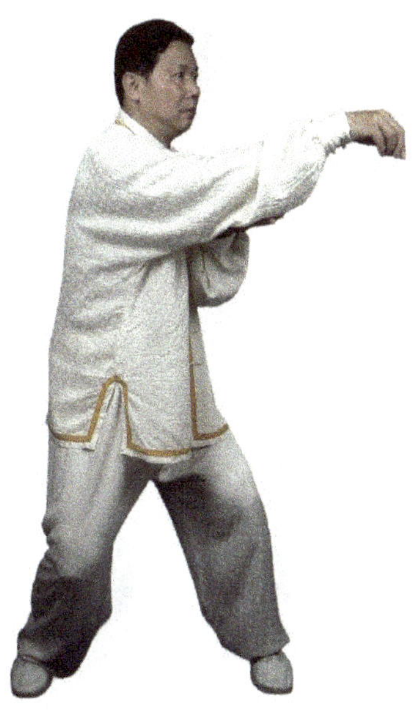

Illustration 16-5 In Stillness Wait for the Movement

3) In Stillness Wait for the Movement

The previous movement pauses slightly, the body slightly turns left, both legs bend at the knees to squat down changing to a horse stance. The right arm revolves inward, the right hand five fingers close together changing to a snake head palm, from the front of the chest turning over to extend, elbows bent, stopping at the front of the head; the left arm revolves outward, the left hand movement is coordinated, returning and stopping below the right elbow, the fingertips point front, the palm faces up. Also at the same time, the Dan Tian sinks inward, breathe in. The tongue rises against the upper palate, the teeth are slightly closed. The eyes look at the right snake head palm, the intention is on sinking elbow joints lower, the breath circulates through the hand Three Yang channels. (Illustration 16-5)

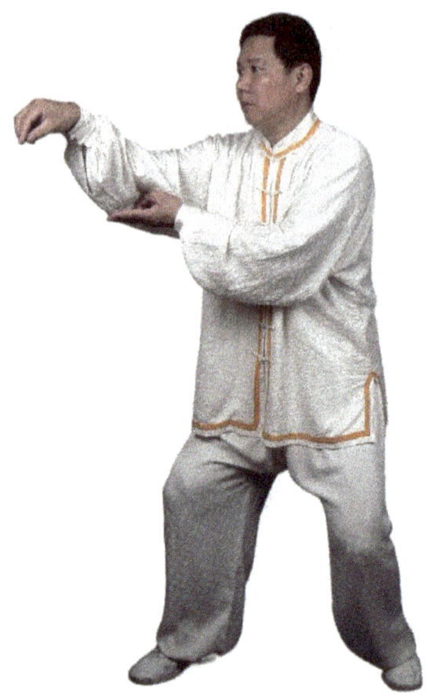

Illustration 16-6 In Stillness Wait for the Movement

The previous movement does not stop, the body turns right, the waist swaying and the upper body hand position does not change, it position of the upper limbs and hands does not change, they follow the turning motion smoothly. At the same time, the Dan Tian sticks outward, breathe out. The tongue is close to the lower palate, the teeth are lightly closed. The eyes follow the turning movement of the right snake head palm, the intention is on quieting the mind and waiting for the movement. (Illustration 16-6)

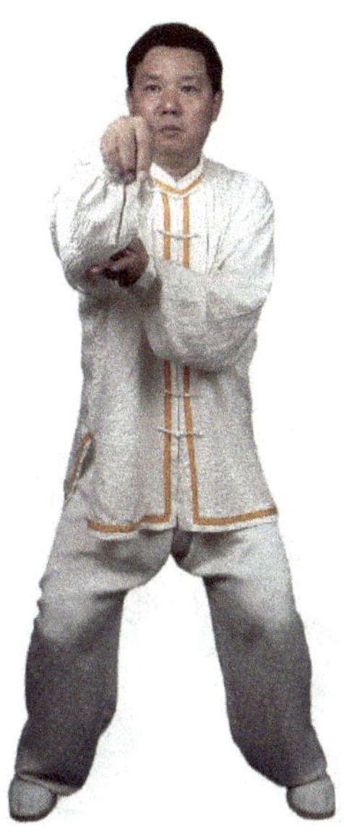

Illustration 16-7 In Stillness Wait for the Movement

The previous movement does not stop, the body sways to the left, both legs gradually straighten. The center of gravity rises with the turning of the body, facing south, naturally standing straight. The movement of the upper body does not change. Also at the same time, the Dan Tian sinks inward, breathe in. The tongue rises against the upper palate, the teeth are slightly closed. The eyes follow the movement of the right palm, the intention is on the Shen Shu acupuncture point, the breath circulates through the Dai Mai. (Illustration 16-7)

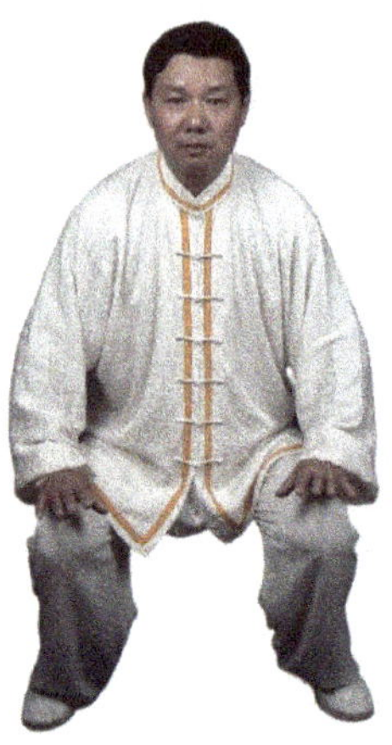

Illustration 16-8 In Stillness Wait for the Movement

The previous movement pauses slightly, both legs bend at the knees to squat down changing to a horse stance. At the same time, both arms revolve inward and both elbows hold together, the hands turn toward the front of the body in an arc shape and press down, stopping in front of the abdomen. The palms face down, the fingertips point forward. At the same time, the Dan Tian sticks outward, breathe out. The tongue rests on the lower palate; the teeth are lightly closed. The eyes look slightly downward; the intention is at the Dan Tian, the breath circulates through both the Du Mai and the Ren Mai. (Illustration 16-8)

4) White Snake Sticks out its Tongue Right Posture

These movement methods are entirely the same as for White Snake Sticks out its Tongue Left posture, but the left and right sides are reversed (see Illustrations 16-1, 16-2, 16-3, 16-4).

5) Gather Inside Return to the Origin

This movement method is entirely the same as for Pushing the Mountain Extremely Empty Initially (see Illustration 2-1). The previous movement does not stop, the next movement method is entirely the same as Extreme Emptiness Exercise, Blend the Elements with one breath (see Illustration 1-8).

Main Points and Functions

In practicing White Snake Sticks out its Tongue exercise, the two fingers move front jab with force, and must be synchronized with the front hand pulling back, like pulling a bow. The whole body must be relaxed, the chest is slightly contained, the body is upright and straight. When collecting the energy and spirit, use the waist to drive the rousing movement of the whole body, the center of gravity it's lowering and swaying of the waist must be simultaneous and connected, when turning the body sink the chest, raise the heels, relax the shoulders, sink the elbow, raise the anus and pull up.

When practicing this exercise method additionally it is necessary to strive for. the three centers must join, the three intentions must link, and the four limbs must be neatly connected. The three centers which must be joined are: the crown center Bai Hui acupuncture point sinking inward, the foot center Yong Quan acupuncture point rising upward, and hand center Lao Gong acupuncture points withdrawing and returning, resulting in the three breaths converging in the Dan Tian. If the crown center does not turn downward, then upper breath cannot flow to the Dan Tian; if the foot center does not rise up, then lower breath cannot return to the Dan Tian; if the hand centers do not withdraw and return, then outer breath cannot return to the Dan Tian. Therefore, it is necessary for the three centers to combine and merge, the breath then can return and gather at one place to refine the golden pill.

The three intentions which must be linked and consistently connected are the mind intention, the inner breath intention, and the strength intention. Of the three intentions, use the mind as the advisor, use the inner breath as the primary commander, and the strength as the soldiers. If the inner breath is not full, then the force will be weak, no matter what is done, it's useless. Therefore, the breath, intention must first be refined, then one can command the strength be sent out, inwardly, to join the mind intention.

The four extremities which must be together are namely the tongue presses, the teeth close, the fingers and toes grip, the pores tighten. When the tongue rises against the upper palate, saliva increases and the qi and blood circulate, when the tongue sinks to the lower palate, the saliva returns to the Dan Tian with the breath out, when the teeth are closed the inner breath can penetrate to the bone marrow, when the fingers and toes close inward, the inner breath can flow through the muscles; the pores are tight. There is no first or last, slow or fast part, if in these places there is one that cannot be done, then it will be easy to becoming angry, scattered, lazy, or to appear to have no energy or spirit.

In the movement raising of the heel, is to gradually let the person who is practicing develop a level of heel breath. Zhuang Zi said: "The true person breathes using the heels, most people breathe using the throat." In a normal person's respiration, everything flows down the throat, returning to the outside of the chest Zhong Wan acupuncture point, it cannot be connected with earlier heaven breath, like a tadpole drinking water in through the mouth and out through the gills. This is Zhuang Zi's so-called "True person breathes using the heels," the heel, the true breath have deep meaning.

It can be said that the breathing of an average person id later heaven breath, the breathing of true person's breath is earlier heaven breath, namely hidden breath circulates the breath can flow straight to the heel. Zhuang Zi said: "The crown gate opening is impressive, the heel of the foot is the key to lively movement. During practice, use the idea of fine and small movements, adjust the breathing, and let go of distracting thoughts.

Also must take this type of thinking activity, gradually reduce to a minimum, then it disappears. The mind becomes empty and quiet, the inner breath naturally flows through the whole body, from the crown of the head Bai Hui, down to the toes and heels. The body center of gravity lowering and the heels rising, can mobilize the foot three yin channels, the foot three yang channels, and also has certain effects on the liver, spleen, and kidneys. At the same time, raising the heels also can increase the whole body extension, thereby having the benefits of strengthening the waist and invigorating the kidneys.

Practice Method

Each time, practice 6 times or 12 times to make one set, practicing again and again in succession is fine. The extent of the movement being larger or smaller, moving higher or lower is without restriction, depending on the age of the person practicing being older or younger, whether the physical strength is greater or lesser, and the weakness or strength in the body.

Acupuncture Points 点穴 (dian xue)

Lao Gong xue 劳宫穴 Palace of Toil PC-8[who]

Bai Hui xue 百会穴 Hundred Convergences GV-20[who]

Yong Quan xue 涌泉穴 Bubbling Spring KC-1[who]

Shen Shu xue 肾俞穴 Kidney BL-23[who]

Dai Mai 带脉 Girdling Vessel GIV, GB-26[who]

Du Mai 督脉 Governing Vessel GV[who]

Ren Mai 任脉 Controlling Vessel; Conception Vessel CV[who]

Zhong Wan xue 中脘穴 Central Stomach Duct CV-12[who]

San Yang jing 三阳经 Three Yang Channels

Set 17 Leopard Climbs a Tree Exercise

Leopard Climbs a Tree, the breath climbs through,

outside and inside, above and below, strength is endless.

Everywhere circulate the kidney breath

to support the human body,

one must also recharge later heaven energy and breath.

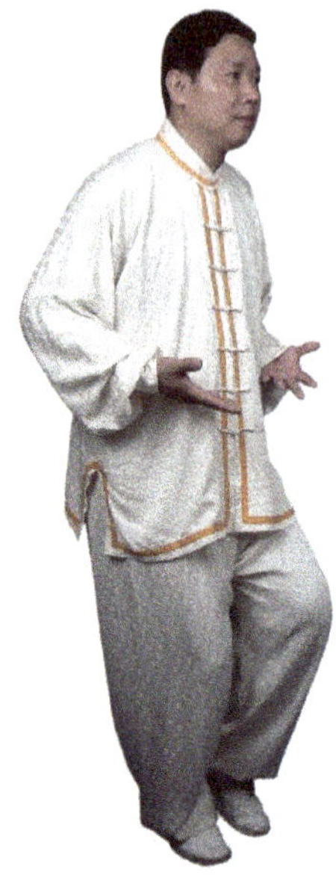

Illustration 17-1 Leopard Climbs a Tree Left Posture

1) Preparation

These movement methods are exactly the same as for Extreme Emptiness Exercise, Preparation Postures. (see Illustrations 1-1, 1-2, 1-3, 1-4)

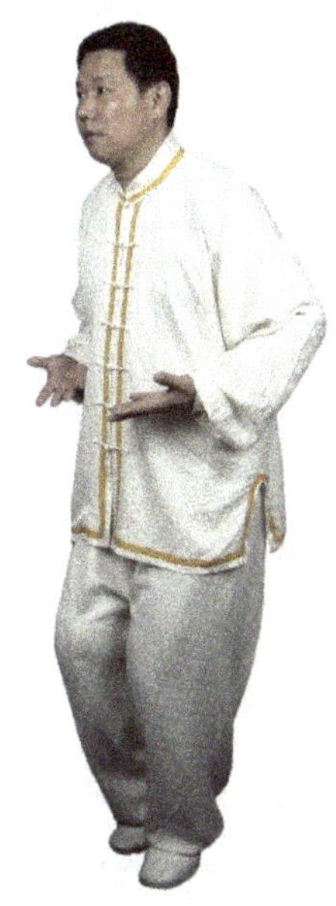

Illustration 17-2 Leopard Climbs a Tree Left Posture

2) Leopard Climbs a Tree Left Posture

The previous movement pauses slightly, the body turns left 45 degrees, the center of gravity shifts to over the right leg, slightly squatting down. The left foot heel rises, the front of the foot stretches straight, the toes slightly close inward, completely empty to rest on the ground, changing to a left high empty stance. Both arms revolve outward, both hands from the sides of the body rising and lifting together in an arc shape, Yang palms stopping at the sides of the chest. The fingertips point front, the palms face up. At the same time, the Dan Tian sinks inward, breathe in. The tongue rises against the upper palate, the teeth are slightly closed. The eyes follow the motion of the body; the intention is on raising the center of the foot Yong Quan acupuncture point. (Illustration 17-1 and 17-2)

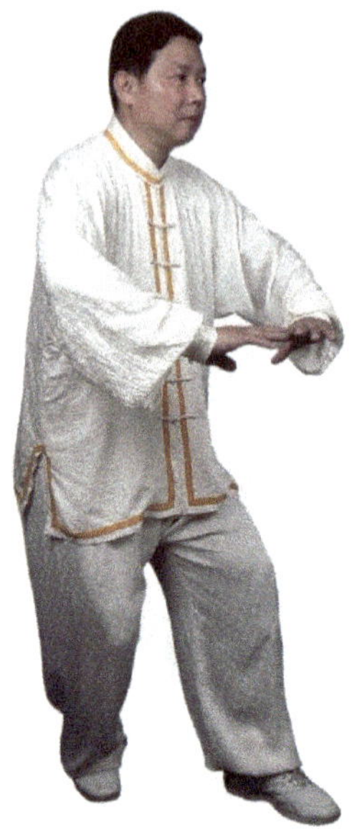

Illustration 17-3 Leopard Climbs a Tree Left Posture

The previous movement does not stop, the body's center of gravity sinks down, the whole left foot is flat on the ground changing to a left four six step, both arms rotate inward, both hands from the front of the chest turn over and press down, at the same height as the abdomen, the fingertips point front, the palms face down and move down. At the same time, the Dan Tian sticks outward, breathe out. The tongue rests on the lower palate, the teeth are lightly closed. The eyes look downward to the front; the intention is on the ends of the spine, sending out strength from the spine. (Illustration 17-3)

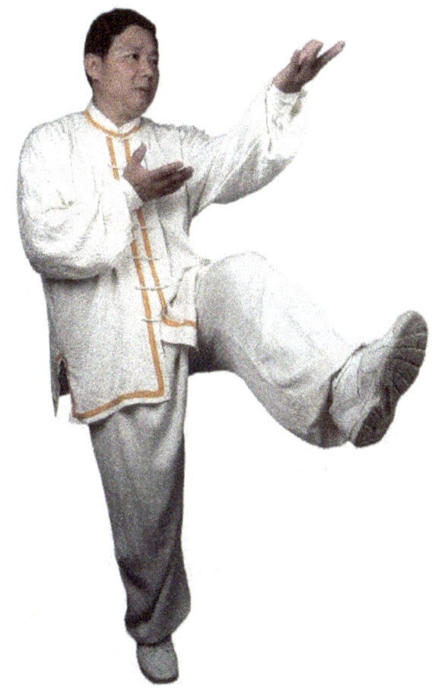

Illustration 17-4 Leopard Climbs a Tree Left Posture

The previous movement pauses slightly, the body's center of gravity shifts backward over the right leg; the left foot toes sway outward and lift up, pressing out briefly at the height of the knee, the toes point toward the upper left, the sole of the foot faces front, changing to left Leopard Rising posture. At the same time, both arms revolve outward, both hands to the front and up pierce out, the left hand is in front and above, at the same height as the throat; the right hand is at the left elbow joint. The fingertips of both hands face front; the centers of the palms face up. Also at the same time, the Dan Tian sinks inward, breathe in. The tongue rises against the upper palate, the teeth are slightly closed. The eyes look toward the left front, the intention is on left foot toe Xia Xi acupuncture point, the breath circulates through the foot's Shao Yang Dan channel. (Illustration 17-4)

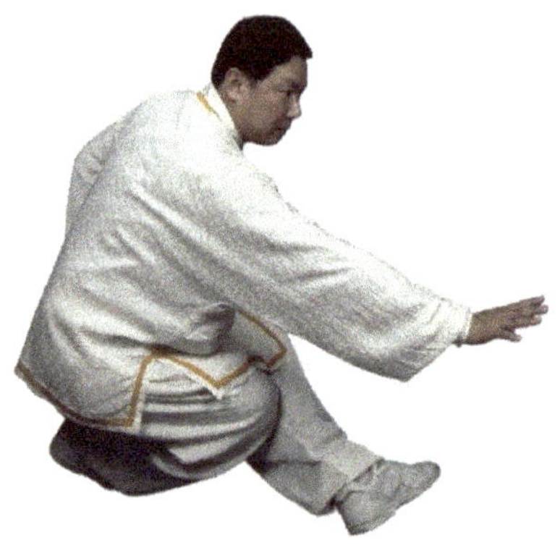

Illustration 17-5 Leopard Climbs a Tree Left Posture

The previous movement does not stop, the body's center of gravity sinks down. The toes of the left foot swing outward to the front and drop down; the right heel leaves the ground, the body slightly inclines forward, the hips sit over the right calf changing into Leopard Left Sinking posture. At the same time, both arms revolve inward, both hands together use strength to split, chop, push, and press down to the front. The left hand drops to the side of the left thigh, the fingertips point front, the palm faces down; the right hand lowers from the navel area, stopping above the left foot, the fingertips point front and up, the palms face front and down. Also at the same time, the Dan Tian sticks outward, breathe out. The tongue rests on the lower palate, the teeth are lightly closed. The eyes look front and down, the intention is on the thigh. (Illustration 17-5)

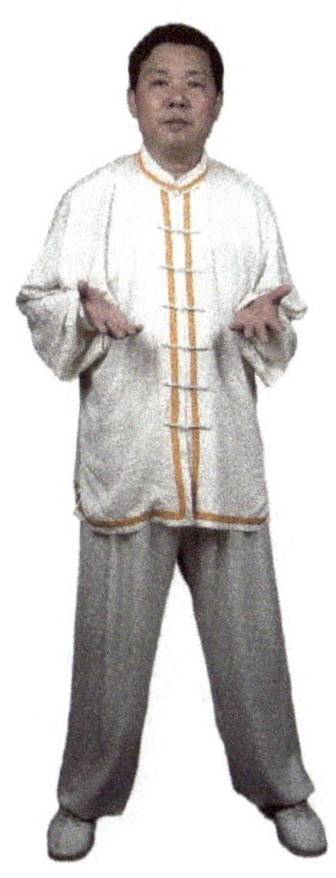

Illustration 17-6 Turn the Body, Small Return

3) Turn the Body, Small Return

The previous movement pauses slightly, the body turns right 45 degrees. The previous movement pauses slightly. After circulating the breath out and in two times, both legs extend to stand naturally. At the same time, both arms revolve to the outside; both hands together turn inward and rise upward, the heels of the palms stop just below both breasts. The fingertips of both hands point front, the palms face up. At the same time, the Dan Tian sinks inward, breathe in. The tongue rises against the upper palate, the teeth are slightly closed, the eyes look to the front. (Illustration 17-6)

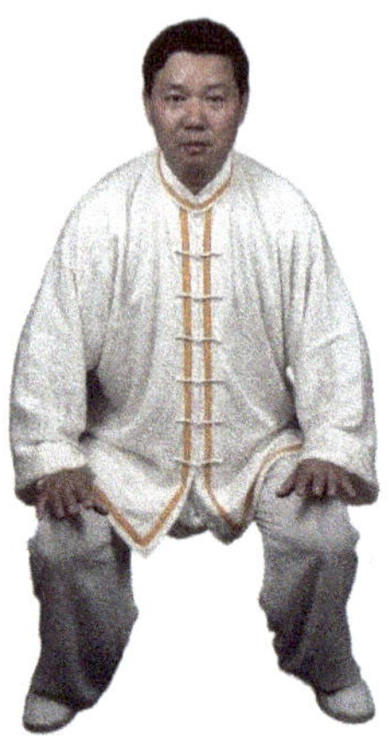

Illustration 17-7 Turn the Body, Small Return

The previous movement does not stop, the body's center of gravity lowers, both legs bend at the knees to squat down changing to a horse stance. At the same time, both arms revolve inward and both elbows hold together, the hands turn toward the front of the body in an arc shape and press down, stopping in front of the abdomen. The palms face down, the fingertips point forward. At the same time, the Dan Tian sticks outward, breathe out. The tongue rests on the lower palate; the teeth are lightly closed. The eyes look slightly downward; the intention is at the Dan Tian, the breath circulates through both the Du Mai and the Ren Mai. (Illustrations 17-7, 17-8)

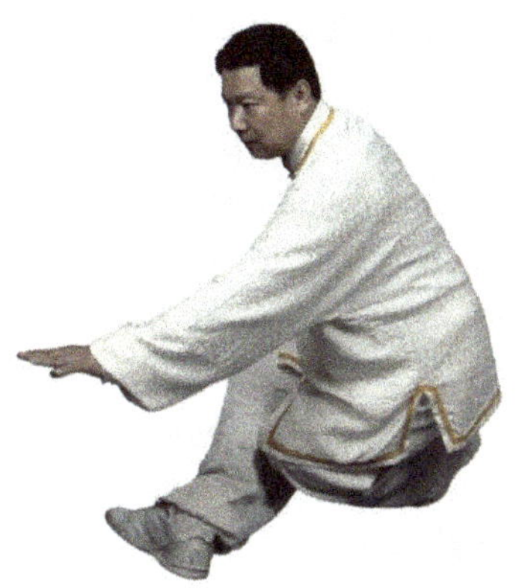

Illustration 17-8 Turn the Body, Small Return

4) Leopard Climbs a Tree Right Posture

These movement methods are entirely the same as for Both Appear Left posture, but the left and right sides are reversed (see Illustrations 17-1, 17-2, 17-3, 17-4, 17-5).

5) Conclude the Set, Return to the Beginning

This movement method is entirely the same as for Pushing the Mountain Extremely Empty Initially (see Illustration 2-1). The previous movement does not stop, the next movement method is entirely the same as Extreme Emptiness Exercise, Blend the Elements with one breath (see Illustration 1-8).

Main Points and Functions

In Leopard Climbs a Tree exercise the stepping out with the leg movement must be at the same time as piercing up with both palms, the feet and palms arrive together, when sinking the nose, feet, and fingertips must be connected with each other, on a vertical plane. The body center of gravity is front three parts, back seven parts. The front foot must extend as straight as possible, the hips must be over the back heel. The waist must sink inward, the head must hold upward, the back knee must set against and behind the front leg knee joint. The tongue must rise upward, send the inner breath downward, the teeth must be gently closed, slightly closed, to make the breath and blood flow and circulate through all the channels, meridians, and acupuncture points in the body. The energy and spirit must be concentrated, use the waist to drive the turning movement of the whole body. The elbows don't leave the ribs, the hands don't leave the center, drill, split, the body moving in, all must be together and in harmony.

A person may regard breath as the foundation, regard mind as the root, regard breathing as the master. One breath out and a hundred meridians all open, one breath in and a hundred meridians all close. Under heaven and earth ten thousand things de cycle of rotation, none put forth these two words, inhale and exhale. This breathing method has three segments rationale and three parts workmanship, namely the criteria for practicing China's Wudang Qigong. The first segment, breathing naturally and freely, having a form on the outside, this is called adjusting the breath, it is also called refining and transforming the breath, the first step of workmanship; the second segment, breathing has a form on the inside, focusing the breathing at the lower Dan Tian, this is called circulating the breath, and is also called "fetal breath," and it is also called refining the breath to transform the spirit the second step of workmanship; in the third section the heart and kidney are joined with the inner breathing, without form without shape, seeming continuous, seeming to exist and not exist, without sound without breath, it is also called refining the spirit and returning to emptiness the third step of workmanship.

In general, when practicing inner breath circulation the requirements are: gentle out, slowly in, breathing through the nose, not using the mouth (except for those with a stuffy nose). At first accumulate true intention and breath with inner breath, gradually extend and fill. Stand straight without leaning, harmonious and not drifting, without form and without appearance.

During practice, the thoughts must achieve the three observations: 1) observe clearly, 2) observe fullness, 3) observe openings. To observe clearly is to observe clearly, it is self-explanatory, with common knowledge then the mind will be peaceful, the spirit lively, the thoughts calm, and in this way can control the passions. To observe fullness, this means the under heaven there is loss and there is increase, receiving not enough, the intention isn't enough, do the hard work to strengthen the breath, in order to seek a long life and see forever; to observe the openings, this means to sincerely observe the rules and requirements, then gradually subdue so that the heart can become settled and calm, the calm then naturally sends out true yang, the temperament naturally improves. After a long time, the spirit and the breath merge, the spirit embryo forms.

Practice Method

Each time, practice 6 times or 12 times to make one set, practicing again and again in succession is fine. The extent of the movement being larger or smaller, moving higher or lower is without restriction, depending on the age of the person practicing being older or younger, whether the physical strength is greater or lesser, and the weakness or strength in the body.

Acupuncture Points 点穴 (dian xue)

Du Mai 督脉 Governing Vessel GV[who]

Ren Mai 任脉 Controlling Vessel; Conception Vessel CV[who]

Yong Quan xue 涌泉穴 Bubbling Spring KC-1[who]

Xia Xi xue 侠溪穴 Pinched Ravine GB-43[who]

Zu Shao Yang Dan jing 足少阳胆经 Foot's Lesser Yang Gallbladder channel GB[who]

Set 18 Peaks Pay Homage to the Top Exercise

Seventy-two peaks pay homage to the golden crown,
Thirty-six cliffs strengthen and replenish (yin) Kun[28]
Refining the Dan Tian results in a long life treasure
that ten thousand measures of yellow gold
cannot offer a person.

---

[28] 坤 (Kun) the Receptive; from the ba gua (eight trigrams)

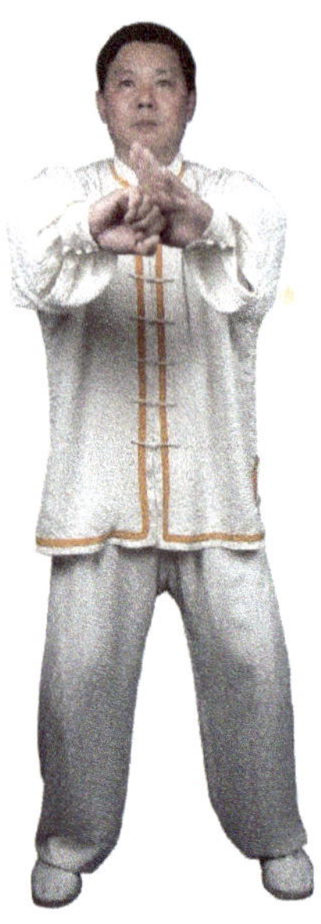

Illustration 18-1 With a Sincere Heart Pay Homage

1) Preparation

These movement methods are exactly the same as for Extreme Emptiness Exercise, Preparation Postures. (see Illustrations 1-1, 1-2, 1-3, 1-4)

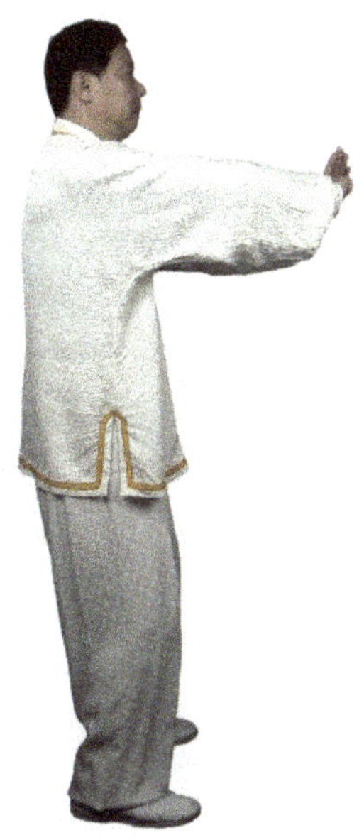

Illustration 18-2 With a Sincere Heart Pay Homage

2) With a Sincere Heart Pay Homage to the Mountain

The previous movement pauses slightly, both arms revolve to the outside, both hands from the sides of the body rise upward and lift, stopping below the lip at the Cheng Jiang acupuncture point, the left palm fingertips point up, the center of the palm faces right; the right palm changes to a fist, leaning against the left palm Lao Gong acupuncture point, the fist is forward and up, the center of the fist faces left. At the same time, the Dan Tian sinks inward, breathe in. The tip of the tongue rises against the upper palate, the teeth are slightly closed. The eyes are slightly closed, the intention is on the crown of the head Bai Hui acupuncture point. (Illustrations 18-1 and 18-2)

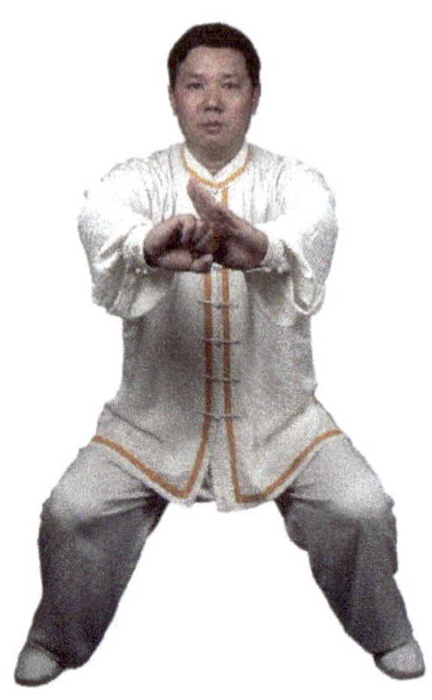

Illustration 18-3 With a Sincere Heart Pay Homage

The previous movement does not stop, both legs bend at the knees to squat down, the body inclines forward. Both knee joints close inward, raise the heels, the elbow joints hold together. Both hands hand positions do not change, then they lower following an arc shape. Also at the same time, the Dan Tian sticks outward, breathe out. The tongue rests on the lower palate, the teeth are lightly closed. The eyes look inside, the intention is on the Dan Tian. (Illustration 18-3)

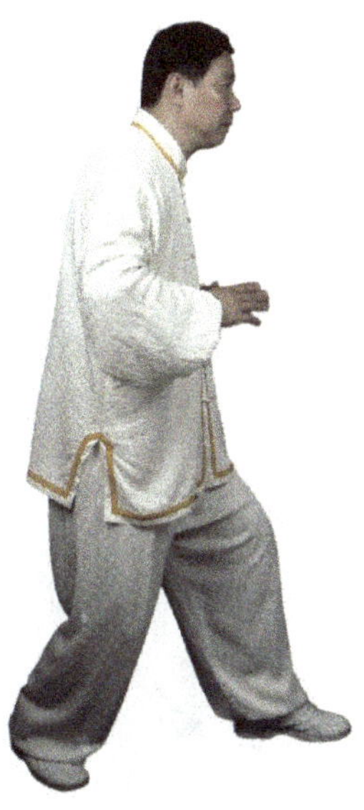

Illustration 18-4 Peaks Pay Homage to the Top Left Posture

3) Peaks Pay Homage to the Summit Left Posture

The previous movement pauses slightly, the body turns left 90 degrees, the center of gravity rises upward, the toes of the right foot close inward, the knees bend slightly to squat down, the left heel is lifted from the ground, the sole of the foot extends flat, the toes point slightly inward and lightly touch the ground, the left knee is slightly bent, the body's center of gravity sinks onto the right leg changing to a left high empty stance. At the same time, both arms revolve inward, both hands from the front of the head lower in the shape of an arc and open in opposite directions, stopping in front of the abdomen. The fingertips face each other; the palms are angled forward and down. At the same time, the Dan Tian sinks inward, breathe in. The tongue rises against the upper palate, the teeth are slightly closed. The eyes follow the turning of the body, the intention is on keeping the shoulders down and sinking the elbows, the breath circulates through the hand Shao Yang San Jiao channel. (Illustration 18-4)

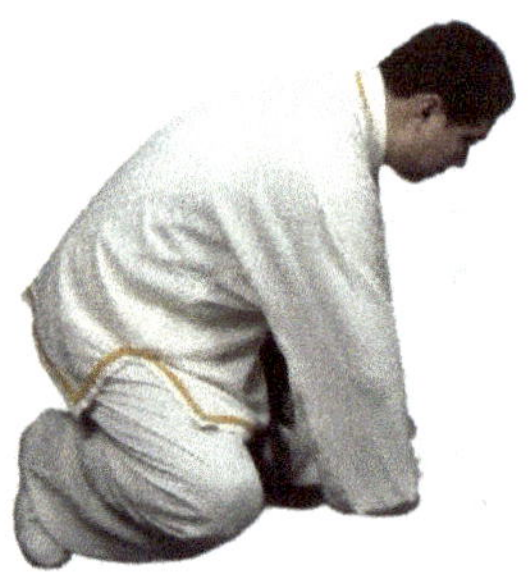

Illustration 18-5 Peaks Pay Homage to the Top Left Posture

The previous movement does not stop, the body's center of gravity moves forward, sinking down over the left leg; the right foot toes remain on the ground, the heel rises. Both legs bend at the knees to completely squat down, the upper body pressing down over the left leg. Both palms face front and push down, stopping in front of the left foot toes, the fingertips face each other, the palms face down and press down to the ground. Also at the same time, the Dan Tian sticks outward, breathe out. The tongue rests on the lower palate, the teeth are lightly closed. The eyes look forward and down, the intention is on raising the right heel, the breath circulates through the foot Tai Yang Pang Guang channel. (Illustration 18-5)

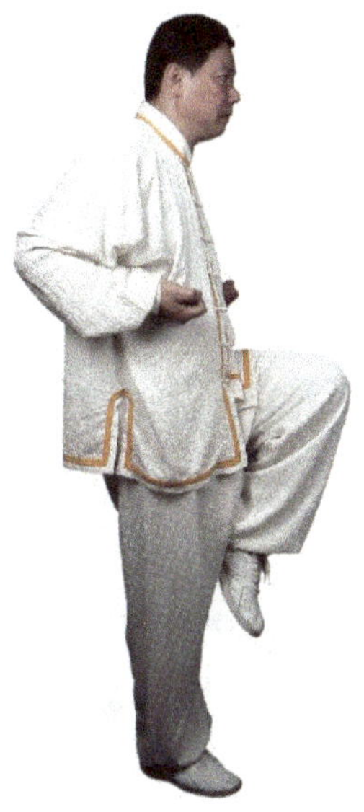

Illustration 18-6 Peaks Pay Homage to the Top Left Posture

The previous movement pauses slightly, the body's center of gravity shifts over the right leg, the right leg straightens, the whole right foot is touching the ground; the left leg bends and rises, the toes point down, the font of the foot extends straight changing to a left single leg standing posture. At the same time, both arms revolve outward, both palms describe an arc in front of the body, stopping at both sides of the Dan Tian. The palms face front, the fingertips point down. At the same time, the Dan Tian sinks inward, breathe in. The tongue rises against the upper palate, the teeth are slightly closed. The eyes look forward, the intention is on the ten fingers closing to grab, the breath circulates through the hand Three Yang channels. (Illustration 18-6)

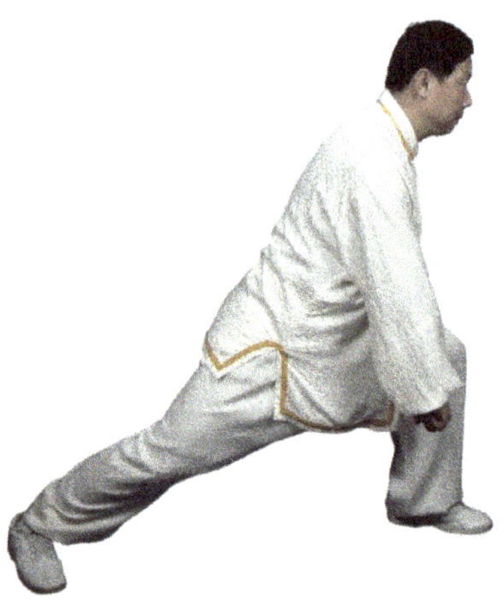

Illustration 18-7 Peaks Pay Homage to the Top Left Posture

The previous movement does not stop, the left foot lowers to the front, the toes slightly close to the inside, the knee bends to half squat; the right leg is firm and the knee straightens, the toes close inward changing to a left bow stance. At the same time, both arms revolve inward, both hands bend, grab, seize, and hold changing into fists to strike down, stopping in front and just below both sides of the left knee joint. The two hands are ten centimeters apart, the palms face inward, the fists face down. At the same time as striking down, the Dan Tian sticks outward, breathe out. The tongue rests on the lower palate, the teeth are lightly closed. The eyes look down at the space between both hands, the intention is on stretching the elbows and urging the inner breath. (Illustration 18-7)

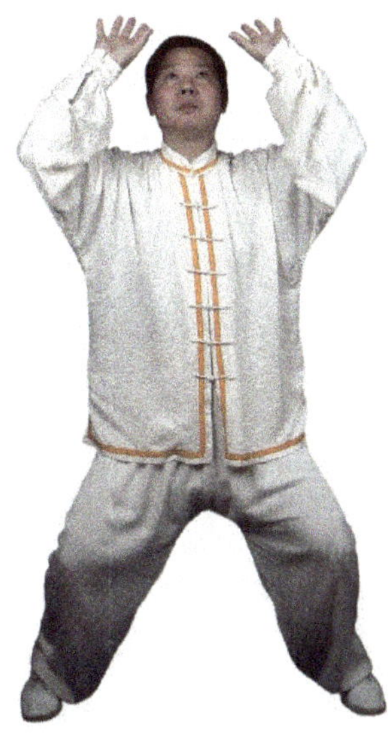

Illustration 18-8 Bow with the Body, Push with the Palms

4) Bow with the Body, Push with the Palms

The previous movement pauses slightly, the body turns right 90 degrees. The body's center of gravity rises smoothly, changing to face the South and naturally stand straight. At the same time, both arms bend at the elbows and press up, both fists change into palms, using the backs of the hands to lead the breath in an arc pressing up, stopping at the forehead. The fingertips point up, the palms face front. At the same time as pressing upward, the Dan Tian sinks inward, breathe in. The tongue rests on the lower palate, the teeth are lightly closed. The eyes look front and up, the intention is on turning over the little finger Shao Chong acupuncture point, the breath circulates through the hand Shao Yin Xin channel. (Illustration 18-8)

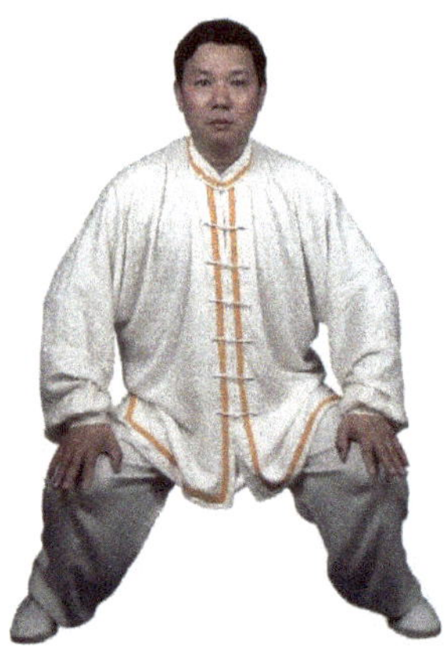

Illustration 18-9 Bow with the Body, Push with the Palms

The previous movement does not stop, both legs bend at the knees to squat down changing to a horse stance. The upper body leans forward, both hands from the forehead press down in an arc shape, stopping at the front of the knee joints. The heels of the palms rest against the tops of the knee caps, the fingertips point down at an angle pointing to the toes. When pressing down, the Dan Tian sticks outward, breathe out. The tongue rests on the lower palate, the teeth are lightly closed. The eyes look front and down, the intention is on the Dan Tian, the breath circulates through the large heavenly circle. (Illustration 18-9)

5) Peaks Pay Homage to the Summit Right Posture

These movement methods are entirely the same as for Group of Peaks Pay Homage to the Summit Left posture, but the left and right sides are reversed. (see Illustrations 18-4, 18-5, 18-6, 18-7)

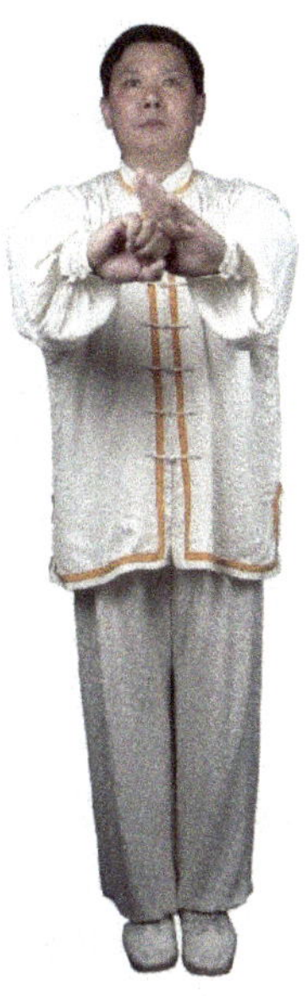

Illustration 18-10 Return to the Beginning

6) Return to the Beginning

The previous movement pauses slightly, the body turns left, facing south. Both arms revolve to the outside, both hands from the sides of the body rise and lift, stopping below the lip at the Cheng Jiang, the left palm fingertips point up and the center of the palm faces right; the right palm changes to a fist, leaning against the center of the left palm Lao Gong acupuncture point, the fist faces up, the center of the palm faces left. Also at the same time, the Dan Tian sinks inward, breathe in. The tongue rises against the upper palate; the teeth are slightly closed. The eyes are slightly closed; the intention is at the crown of the head the Bai Hui acupuncture point. Then, both hands lower, to stop at the sides of the body and change to a standing straight posture. (Illustration 18-10)

Main Points and Functions

During practice, the foot step forward, space of the step, rising and falling all must with the hand movements, yin palm, yang palm, arc shape, rotation movements coordinated and connected, also must use the waist as the governor of the movement, raising up the back, shoulders, elbows, hands, fingers, driving down the hips, knees, feet, and toes. So it is said: "One branch moves, one hundred branches sway" this is true. In Paying Homage to the Peaks Exercise strive to focus on the breathing, supplemented by guiding and leading, pressing to cultivate inner strength workmanship.

The early teachers in refinement, paid attention to the functions of breath in the human body, considering that for heaven and earth, for ten thousand things, none do not need breath, all rely on it to survive. So it is said: "Breath gathers then life, breath disperses then death." A person who wants to live a long life, must love inner breath, nourish inner breath, respect the spirit mind, pay attention to the energy. A person who is good at practicing inside can strengthen the body, outside can dispel evil and resist disease. When moving the inner breath, try to solidify the spirit and clear away worries, concentrate the breath and extend softly, the breathing out and in, achieving: light, relaxed, even, long, deep.

- Light, the respiration is fine and careful.
- Relaxed, the coming and going of the breath is relaxed.
- Even, the rhythm of respiration is well-distributed.
- Long, the time between breathing out and breathing in is longer.
- Deep, the breath penetrates entering the lungs, internal organs, and hundred vessels, unifying the whole body.

The method of refining the golden pill, comes from ancient alchemy. Originally, it referred to smelting ore in a cauldron to make a medicine, to manufacture a "long life never get old" preserve the health wonder-medicine. Later, Taoists called this practice refining the "outer field." And after that, they taught the human body can imitate a cauldron, by refining and nourishing the energy, breath, spirit, can be used as medicines to refine the inner center. The ancients said: "The three best medicines, spirit, breath, and energy, indistinct, mysterious, deep and profound." Energy, breath, spirit although they are called a pill for refining the internal center, but the arrangement and order is different.

"Spirit" serves as ruler and is master. "Energy, breath" serve as ministers and are guests. Ten thousand spirits become one spirit, ten thousand breaths become one breath, with one, ten thousand are created, and ten thousand are returned to one, all created from my "spirit." So then, throughout all of the exercises of Wudang Qigong, all use "spirit" to receive breath, use "spirit" to refine energy, always never separate from "spirit," since "spirit" is the master, "breath is the driving force, and "energy is the foundation. These three in a person's life are the three primary elements, mutually connecting with and using each other. The ancients said: "When the mind is empty, the spirit can congeal, when the spirit congeals the breath gathers, when the breath gathers energy is born." After that, through a process of workmanship, refining, combining and cultivating, one can progressively rejuvenate the material foundation. Zhang the Immortal in the "Awaken Truth Poem" said: "Each person originally has long life medicine, each one may lose it or merely it cast aside. When sweet dew falls, heaven and earth join, yellow sprouts are born in a place that is not separate but joined. A well frog should say it doesn't have a dragon's den, a hedge sparrow is tranquil not knowing the phoenix's nest. The golden pill ripens naturally to fill the room with gold, why is there a need for grass to study cooking cogon grass?"[29] This means that every human

---

[29] cogon grass is a coarse tall grass used for thatching; also used in cooking

body has a long life golden medicine, unfortunately not everyone understands the treasure and in vain casts it aside or misses it entirely. Yin and yang combine with each other, energy and spirit are refined together, the human body's life and metabolism primary elements can be reborn. "Sweet dew" refers to earlier heaven breath, from a clay ball sinking down into the Dan Tian “Golden Sprout” above and below connected, solidifying and gathering becoming a “sage embryo,” this is known as ripening the golden pill. “A room full of gold," then, points to: the one practicing having attained, energy, breath, spirit the three flowers gathered together at the top, the heart, liver, spleen, lungs, kidneys, five breaths return to their original state.

Practice Method

Each time, practice 6 times or 12 times to make one set, practicing again and again in succession is fine. The extent of the movement being larger or smaller, moving higher or lower is without restriction, depending on the age of the person practicing being older or younger, whether the physical strength is greater or lesser, and the weakness or strength in the body.

Acupuncture Points 点穴 (dian xue)

Cheng Jiang xue 承浆穴 Sauce Receptacle CV-24[who]

Lao Gong xue 劳宫穴 Palace of Toil PC-8[who]

Bai Hui xue 百会穴 Hundred Convergences GV-20[who]

Shou Shao Yang San Jiao jing 手少阳三焦经 Hand's Lesser Yang Triple Burner channel TB[who]

Zu Tai Yang Pangguang jing 足太阳膀胱经 Foot's Greater Yang Bladder channel BL[who]

Shao Chong xue 少冲穴 Lesser Thoroughfare HT-9[who]

Shou Shao Yin Xin jing 手少阴心经 Hand's Lesser Yin Heart channel HT[who]

Shou San Yang jing 手三阳经 Hand Three Yang Channels

Notes on the Translation

For those of you thoughtfully reading this work, we would like to start by apologizing for the inevitable mistakes and any misunderstanding they may cause. It has been very difficult to communicate many of the subtleties of the original Chinese in the English version. Part of this responsibility lies with the choices we had to make in translating this book; but part also lies in the differences between the two languages. There are some things English does well; others it does awkwardly. The same is true for Chinese. We made many choices in our word selections. We believe they were the best ones possible. We hope have gained enough understanding through this process to make better ones next time.

We had several ideas in mind while translating this book. These served as our guide in making these choices. We wanted to include the terms and concepts as they are commonly known in the west but we also wanted to be consistent. This resulted in all untranslated names being rendered in standard pinyin. We wanted to be as accurate as possible in translating certain terms, especially those with philosophical implications. This resulted in a quite literal translation. We wanted to keep as close to the original tone and rhythm as possible. This resulted in what we hope is a single voice in both languages.

There are those who would (and did) say we should use a more "natural" voice in the English; with more common structures and patterns. But then the translation would not parallel the original. There are those who said we should simplify some of the sentences and concepts to make them easier to grasp, but then we wouldn't be translating, and in the process, watering-down the meaning. We have tried to include every concept, every idea, particularly in those sections which have philosophical discussions. Where the text describes movement, we have kept the long sentences from the original. In many cases, descriptions of simultaneous movements are long, containing several elements all occurring at the same time. While these could have been broken down into a choppy series of sentences, that would betray both the original text and the intent of the movement to be simultaneous and continuous. Our overall goal was and is to provide an accurate, correct translation. If some of the concepts are abstruse, if some of the ideas are hard to grasp, if some of the symbolism is obscure, this is because they are difficult even for a native Chinese speaker reading the text in the original Chinese.

The short poems at the beginning of each of the 18 exercises were the most difficult to translate. They express the essence, the core purpose or focus of the exercise. In doing so, they use metaphors and symbols. But even though the metaphors and symbols are often explained following the exercise, there are many opportunities for confusion. We hope we have at least come close to capturing some of the imagery from the original.

Prof. Yuzeng Liu
Terri Morgan

June 1999

Acupuncture Points

Set 1 Extreme Emptiness Exercise

Lao Gong xue 劳宫穴 Palace of Toil PC-8[who]

Yong Quan xue 涌泉穴 Bubbling Spring KC-1[who]

Tan Zhong xue 膻中穴 Chest Center CV-17[who]

Jue Yin Gan jing 厥阴肝经 Reverting Yin Liver channel

Xuan Guan qiao 玄关窍 Mysterious Gate (upper Dan Tian)

Bai Hui xue 百会穴 Hundred Convergences GV-20[who]

Qi Hai 气海 Sea of Qi CV-6[who]

Set 2 Pushing the Mountain Exercise

Zhen Yuan 真元 True Breath.

Yuan Qi 元气 Original Breath

Du Mai 督脉 Governing Vessel GV[who]

Ren Mai 任脉 Controlling Vessel; Conception Vessel CV[who]

Hui Yin 会阴 Meeting of Yin (perineum) CV-1[who]

Set 3 Wild Goose Flying Exercise

Zhang Men xue 章门穴 Camphorwood Gate LV-13

Lao Gong xue 劳宫穴 Palace of Toil PC-8[who]

Xuan Guan qiao 玄关窍 Mysterious Gate (upper Dan Tian)

Du Mai 督脉 Governing Vessel GV[who]

Bai Hui xue 百会穴 Hundred Convergences GV-20[who]

Qu Chi xue 曲池穴 Pool at the Bend LI-11[who]

Yong Quan xue 涌泉穴 Bubbling Spring KC-1[who]

Set 4 Bending Crane Exercise

Lao Gong xue 劳宫穴 Palace of Toil PC-8[who]

San Li xue 三里 Three Li ST-36

Nei Guan 内关 Inner Pass PC-6[who]

Wai Guan 外关 Outer Pass TB-5

Zhong Chong 中冲 Central Hub PC-9[who]

Jue Yin Xin Bao jing 厥阴心包经 Reverting Yin Pericardium channel PC[who]

Bai Hui xue 百会穴 Hundred Convergences GV-20[who]

Set 5 Supporting Heaven Exercise

Du Mai 督脉 Governing Vessel GV[who]

Ren Mai 任脉 Controlling Vessel; Conception Vessel CV[who]

Shen Feng xue 神封穴 Spirit Seal KI-23[who]

Lao Gong xue 劳宫穴 Palace of Toil PC-8[who]

Xuan Guan qiao 玄关窍 Mysterious Gate (upper Dan Tian)

Shen Ting xue 神庭穴 Spirit Court GV-24[who]

Hua Gai xue 华盖 Florid Canopy CV-20[who]

Shao Ze xue 少泽 Lesser Marsh SI-1[who]

Da Yang Xiao Chang jing 太阳小肠经 Greater Yang Small Intestine Channel

Yong Quan xue 涌泉穴 Bubbling Spring KC-1[who]

Bai Hui xue 百会穴 Hundred Convergences GV-20[who]

Weilu guan 尾闾关 Coccyx gate

Lulu guan 辘轳关 Winch gate

Yu Zhen 玉枕 Jade Pillow BK-9[who]

Shan Zhong 膻中 (middle Dan Tian)

Set 6 Both Appear Exercise

Du Mai 督脉 Governing Vessel GV[who]

Ren Mai 任脉 Controlling Vessel; Conception Vessel CV[who]

Qi Men xue 期门 Cycle Gate LV-14

Yong Quan xue 涌泉穴 Bubbling Spring KC-1[who]

Lao Gong xue 劳宫穴 Palace of Toil PC-8[who]

Shou Tai Yin Fei jing 手太阴肺经 Hand's Greater Yin Lung channel LU[who]

Hui Yin 会阴 Meeting of Yin (perineum) CV-1[who]

Que Qiao 鹊桥 Bird Bridge

Weilu guan 尾闾关 Coccyx gate

Yao Yang guan 腰阳关 Lumbar Pass GV-3[who]

Ming Men xue 命门穴 Life Gate GV-4[who]

Yin Jiao 阴交 Yin Intersection CV-7[who]

Qi Hai 气海 Sea of Qi CV-6[who]

Set 7 Four Directions Exercise

Du Mai 督脉 Governing Vessel GV[who]

Ren Mai 任脉 Controlling Vessel; Conception Vessel CV[who]

Chong Mai 冲脉 Thoroughfare Vessel; Penetrating Vessel PV

Bai Hui xue 百会穴 Hundred Convergences GV-20[who]

Yong Quan xue 涌泉穴 Bubbling Spring KC-1[who]

Lao Gong xue 劳宫穴 Palace of Toil PC-8[who]

Set 8 Ward Off and Pull Down Exercise

Du Mai 督脉 Governing Vessel GV[who]

Ren Mai 任脉 Controlling Vessel; Conception Vessel CV[who]

Lao Gong xue 劳宫穴 Palace of Toil PC-8[who]

Yong Quan xue 涌泉穴 Bubbling Spring KC-1[who]

Shou Yang Ming Dachang jing 手阳明大肠经 Hand's Yang Brightness Large Intestine channel LI[who]

Shuidao xue 水道穴 Waterway ST-28[who]

Zu Yang Ming Wei Jing 足阳明胃经 Foot's Yang Brightness Stomach channel ST[who]

Shang Yang xue 商阳穴 Shang Yang LI-1[who]

Dai Mai 带脉 Girdling Vessel GIV, GB-26[who]

Chong Mai 冲脉 Thoroughfare Vessel; Penetrating Vessel PV

Set 9 Pipa Exercise

Du Mai 督脉 Governing Vessel GV[who]

Ren Mai 任脉 Controlling Vessel; Conception Vessel CV[who]

Lao Gong xue 劳宫穴 Palace of Toil PC-8[who]

Bai Hui xue 百会穴 Hundred Convergences GV-20[who]

Si Bai xue 四白穴 Four Whites ST-2[who]

Qi Hai 气海 Sea of Qi CV-6[who]

Set 10 Shaking the Tail Feathers Exercise

Du Mai 督脉 Governing Vessel GV[who]

Ren Mai 任脉 Controlling Vessel; Conception Vessel CV[who]

Bai Hui xue 百会穴 Hundred Convergences GV-20[who]

Shao Chong xue 少冲穴 Lesser Thoroughfare HT-9[who]

Lao Gong xue 劳宫穴 Palace of Toil PC-8[who]

Mai Men 脉门 Vessel Gate, Lesser Thoroughfare HT-9[who]

Yong Quan xue 涌泉穴 Bubbling Spring KC-1[who]

Set 11 White Ape Presents Fruit Exercise

Lao Gong xue 劳宫穴 Palace of Toil PC-8[who]

Dai Mai 带脉 Girdling Vessel GIV, GB-26[who]

Zu Shao Yang Dan jing 足少阳胆经 Foot's Lesser Yang Gallbladder channel GB[who]

Cheng Jiang xue 承浆穴 Sauce Receptacle CV-24[who]

Yong Quan xue 涌泉穴 Bubbling Spring KC-1[who]

Shou Tai Yin Fei jing 手太阴肺经 Hand's Greater Yin Lung channel LU[who]

Jue Yin Xinbao jing 厥阴心包经 Reverting Yin Pericardium channel PC[who]

Yu Tang xue 玉堂穴 Jade Hall CV-18[who]

Xuan Guan qiao 玄关窍 Mysterious Gate opening (upper Dan Tian)

Set 12 Red Phoenix Faces the Sun Exercise

Nei Guan 内关 Inner Pass PC-6[who]

Da Ling xue 大陵穴 Great Mound PC-7[who]

Zhou Rong xue 周荣穴 All-Round Flourishing SP-20[who]

Bai Hui xue 百会穴 Hundred Convergences GV-20[who]

Tai Yin Pi jing 太阴脾经 Greater Yin Spleen channel SP[who]

Wai Guan 外关 Outer Pass TB-5

Da Ling xue 大陵穴 Great Mound PC-7[who]

Zhou Rong xue 周荣穴 All-Round Flourishing SP-20[who]

Tai Yin Pi jing 太阴脾经 Greater Yin Spleen channel SP[who]

Lao Gong xue 劳宫穴 Palace of Toil PC-8[who]

Hui Yin 会阴 Meeting of Yin (perineum) CV-1[who]

Yong Quan xue 涌泉穴 Bubbling Spring KC-1[who]

Ming Men xue 命门穴 Life Gate GV-4[who]

Jia Ji xue 夹脊穴 Paravertebrals

Yu Zhen 玉枕 Jade Pillow BK-9[who]

Feng Fu xue 风府穴 Wind House GV-16[who]

Ren Zhong xue 人中穴 Human Center GV-26[who]

Cheng Jiang xue 承浆穴 Sauce Receptacle CV-24[who]

Ren Mai 任脉 Controlling Vessel; Conception Vessel CV[who]

Chang Qiang xue 长强穴 Long and Rigid GV-1[who]

Set 13 Stir the Grass to Seek the Snake Exercise

Lao Gong xue 劳宫穴 Palace of Toil PC-8[who]

Ji Quan xue 极泉穴 Highest Spring HT-1[who]

Bai Hui xue 百会穴 Hundred Convergences GV-20[who]

Kong Zui 孔最 Collection Hole LU-6[who]

Shou Tai Yin Fei jing 手太阴肺经 Hand's Greater Yin Lung Channel LU[who]

Shen Men xue 神门穴 Spirit Gate HT-7[who]

Shou Yang Ming Dachang Jing 手阳明大肠经 Hand's Yang Brightness Large Intestine channel LI[who]

Du Mai 督脉 Governing Vessel GV[who]

Ren Mai 任脉 Controlling Vessel; Conception Vessel CV[who]

Set 14 Dragon and Tiger Join Together Exercise

Du Mai 督脉 Governing Vessel GV[who]

Ren Mai 任脉 Controlling Vessel; Conception Vessel CV[who]

Zhong Ting xue 中庭穴 Center Palace CV-16[who]

Shang Yang xue 商阳穴 Shang Yang LI-1[who]

Shou Yang Ming Dachang jing 手阳明大肠经 Hand's Yang Brightness Large Intestine channel LI[who]

Cheng Jiang xue 承浆穴 Sauce Receptacle CV-24[who]

Ren Zhong xue 人中穴 Human Center GV-26[who]

Xuan Guan qiao 玄关窍 Mysterious Gate opening (upper Dan Tian)

Set 15 Coiling Snake Exercise

Du Mai 督脉 Governing Vessel GV[who]

Ren Mai 任脉 Controlling Vessel; Conception Vessel CV[who]

Yong Quan xue 涌泉穴 Bubbling Spring KC-1[who]

Shen Shu xue 肾俞穴 Kidney BL-23[who]

Zu Tai Yang Pang Guang jing 足太阳膀胱经 Foot's Greater Yang Bladder channel BL[who]

Set 16 White Snake Sticks out its Tongue Exercise

Lao Gong xue 劳宫穴 Palace of Toil PC-8[who]

Bai Hui xue 百会穴 Hundred Convergences GV-20[who]

Yong Quan xue 涌泉穴 Bubbling Spring KC-1[who]

Shen Shu xue 肾俞穴 Kidney BL-23[who]

Dai Mai 带脉 Girdling Vessel GIV, GB-26[who]

Du Mai 督脉 Governing Vessel GV[who]

Ren Mai 任脉 Controlling Vessel; Conception Vessel CV[who]

Zhong Wan xue 中脘穴 Central Stomach Duct CV-12[who]

San Yang jing 三阳经 Three Yang Channels

Set 17 Leopard Climbs a Tree Exercise

Du Mai 督脉 Governing Vessel GV[who]

Ren Mai 任脉 Controlling Vessel; Conception Vessel CV[who]

Yong Quan xue 涌泉穴 Bubbling Spring KC-1[who]

Xia Xi xue 侠溪穴 Pinched Ravine GB-43[who]

Zu Shao Yang Dan jing 足少阳胆经 Foot's Lesser Yang Gallbladder channel GB[who]

Set 18 Peaks Pay Homage to the Top Exercise

Cheng Jiang xue 承浆穴 Sauce Receptacle CV-24[who]

Lao Gong xue 劳宫穴 Palace of Toil PC-8[who]

Bai Hui xue 百会穴 Hundred Convergences GV-20[who]

Shou Shao Yang San Jiao jing 手少阳三焦经 Hand's Lesser Yang Triple Burner channel TB[who]

Zu Tai Yang Pangguang jing 足太阳膀胱经 Foot's Greater Yang Bladder channel BL[who]

Shao Chong xue 少冲穴 Lesser Thoroughfare HT-9[who]

Shou Shao Yin Xin jing 手少阴心经 Hand's Lesser Yin Heart channel HT[who]

Shou San Yang jing 手三阳经 Hand Three Yang Channels

List of Illustrations

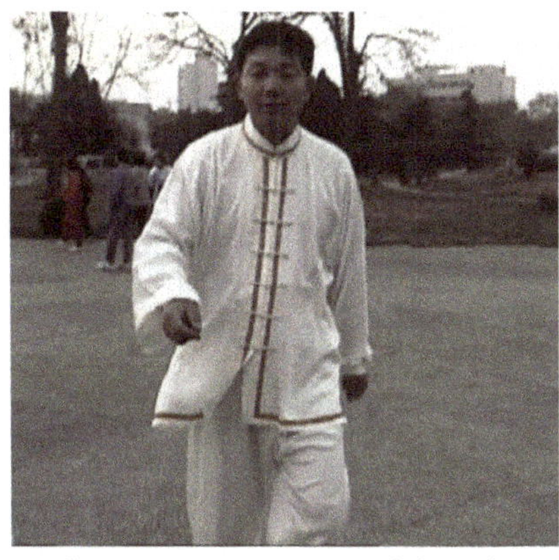

Professor Yuzeng Liu at People's Park in Zhengzhou, 1999

About the Author: Professor Yuzeng Liu began learning Shaolin martial arts from his grandfather when he was six years old. When he was twelve, his shifu, Wang Xixiao, planned for him to inherit Wudang Boxing. Yuzeng Liu is a member of the 31st Generation of disciples of China's Songshan Shaolin Temple, and is famous in the modern generation of China's Songshan Shaolin martial artists, being listed in the 1999 International Directory of Distinguished Leadership. He has compiled and published 13 specialized books on martial arts, and has written more than 100 articles and treatises which have been published in China's public magazines. Professor Liu lives and works in China's ancient Yin Shang dynasty capital city -- Zhengzhou, in Henan province.

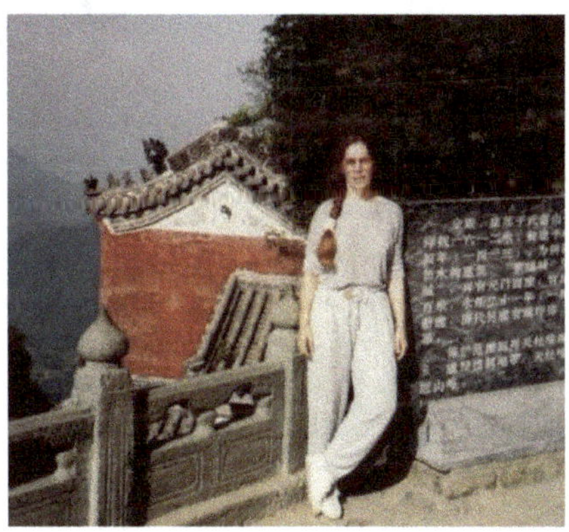

Terri Morgan at Wudangshan, 1995

About the Translator: Terri Morgan started studying Yang style taijiquan in 1985 with Weilun Huang. She won first place at the US championships in Houston in 1989. In 1990 she went to China to teach English. While there, she met Professor Yuzeng Liu and began learning Wudang internal boxing, Xingyi, Bagua, and Sword methods from him. A native of Kansas City, Ms. Morgan received her BA in English from UMKC. In 1995, she was listed in the World Who's Who of Women. She has worked in technlogy for most of her professional career, producing dozens of software manuals and technical articles. Ms. Morgan developed and maintains the Wudang Research Association, the company website, and company publications.

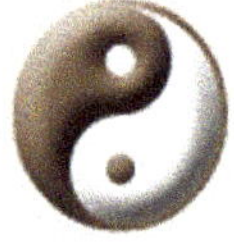

Wudang Research Association

武当气功

第二版

中国

武当山

道家气功

刘玉增著

刘玉增和特丽摩根翻译

第一版

汉语部从武当气功

英语翻译

照片

第一版出版 1999 年
ISBN 0-9672889-0-8

第二版

照片

新的翻译还修改

第二版出版 2023 年
ISBN-13: 978-0-9672889-8-7
ISBN-10: 0-9672889-8-3

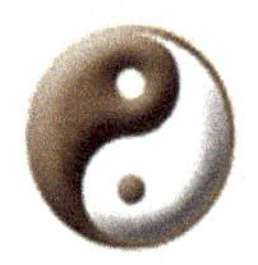

武当研究会

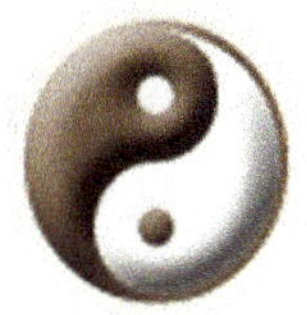

现在将《武当气功》奉献给

全世界的气功、武术的爱好者，与大家结个

善缘。愿大家顺利、平安、長壽。

武当气功

目录

武当气功

前言

中国武当山道家气功因源于武当山[1] 而得 名。武当山又名参上山、太和山，是中国道家 发源圣地之一。素有"寰古无双胜景，天下第 一仙山"、"北重少林"、"南尊武当，之美称。

武当气功将人体拟作"炉鼎，以炼养体 内的精、气、神，为内升。以意运气，以气催身，凝神净虑，抱无守一。可以使练习者祛病 强身，延年宜寿；运五行八法之气，可以抗邪 防暴。真乃内以养生，外以祛恶，内外兼修，独树一帜的练气方法。

相传东汉阴长生、晋谢允、唐吕洞宾、明 张三丰皆修炼于此山[2]，"张三丰擅辟谷[3]" 是当时颇受羣众欢迎的道士。[4]

现将根据武当气功家王希孝师父[5] 亲授的 武当气功、气功秘抄本和有关道家养性、炼气 的资料整理编写的《武当气功》 书，献绐诸 位同好。由于武当气功功法甚多，难以全部收 录，恳请海内外气功高手发掘、整理、补充，使之逐步完善。

本书在编写过程中，武当山武当拳法研究 会秘书长黄学文给予关注和支持，龙得到了河 南公安高尊专科学校、河南

---

[1] 武当山位于湖北省西北部均县境内。漠武帝时始置武当县，属河南南阳郡。

[2] 见《宗教词典》625 页 "武当山命。 "

[3] 辟谷：一种养生修炼，祛谷食气的练功方法。

[4] 见《道教史》262 页。

[5] 王希孝师父：河南洛阳孟津人，幼随王宗岳祖师五代传人习练太极拳。后遵师命上 武当山，从师李合起道长。解放后回归故里，乃我祖父刘文周公之契友，后在郑州市 人民公圉设场授徙。

省体育报刊社、河 南前衛气功联合会、郑州市武协武当拳法研究 会。以及诸位好友和弟子们的大力协助，谨致 谢意。

本书在翻译过程中，得到了美国国际武当 内家拳研究会的全力协助。十分感谢！

刘玉增

1999 年 6 月 28 日

武当气功

中国

武当山

道家气功

第一章　概述

道家气功以无极、推山、雁飞、鹤坳、托天、两仪、四象、棚捋、琵琶、抖翎、献果、朝阳、拨草、龙虎、蛇盘、吐芯、上树、朝顶 18 种练功方法组成。练习道家气功，以个人单练、教师指导为主，按照呼吸、息调、调息、胎息等内气运行法则，进行坐、卧、行、收等功法研练。

第一步为内气运行小周天，亦称谓头关，叫做炼精化气。合精、气、神为神气。第二步为内气运行大周天，亦称谓中关，叫做炼气化神。和神气为神。第三步为万物合为一殊，亦谓炼神还虚复归于无极，明心见性壮身延年。

精、气、神，指人体先天的元精、元气、元神。其中精为基础，气是动力，神为主宰。以神驭气，以神炼精。人体精固则气充，神足则精力充沛，身心健康。反之，则精虚气竭，气竭则神逝。因此，在炼养过程中，时刻重视养精蓄锐，调气摄神。精满则气壮，气壮则神旺，神旺则体健、病祛。

武当气功

老子《道德经．三章》："虚其心、实其腹。弱其至、强其骨"乃是练习中国道家气功的座右铭。学习一种功法，要懂得一种功法，精熟一种功法。一种练习道家气功的方法没有学会，暂时不要练习另一种练功方法。一式动作不会，专攻此式，不可习练它式。不可好高骛远，要虚心、有恒，内外兼修，逐步达到腹内轻松气腾然，气以直养而无害。丹田充盈，内气畅通无阻，气、力由脊背而发，随心所欲。专一，求实，练习不懈，持之以恒，循规蹈矩，炼气养体，修心养性，以求空静、无为，而长寿。

第二章 道家气功之妙用

中国道家气功，古时候称谓导引、吐纳、炼气、炼丹、坐观、辟谷，或叫内功。很早就在人民群众中广泛流传，1973 年中国湖南长沙马王堆西汉墓中出土的帛画《导引图》中，计有 44 幅姿势不同的炼气动作；古代名医华佗曾传授吴晋以“五禽之戏”，作为健身祛病长寿之运动。庄子曰：“吐故纳新，熊经鸟伸也。导引之士，养形之人也。”经常练习中国道家气功功法，炼养内气，则谷气消，血脉通，不生病，人尤户枢不朽是也。千百年的实践证明，练习道家气功，对防病、治病、健体长寿都起着极其重要的作用。

第一节 对呼吸系统的作用

呼吸系统的机能，是吸收外界的氧气，排出体内的二氧化碳，保证体内新陈代谢的正常进行。练习道家气功时，采用特殊呼吸方式，如逆式呼吸、喉头呼吸、丹田呼吸等，以引起五脏六腑的活动，而消耗大量的能量，这就促使呼吸器官要加倍地工作，吸入大量的氧气（也就是清气），同时也排出大量的二氧化碳（也就是浊气），从而使它受到了很好的锻炼。尤其是练习了“气沉丹田”这种横膈肌运动的呼吸方式，已在医疗保健工作和全民健身运动中起到了很好的效应。

呼吸系统机能的提高，主要表现在胸廓活动范围加大，肺活量增加。一般入深吸气时的胸围比呼气时大 7-9 厘米，肺活量为 3500 毫升左右。而经常练习中国道家-道家气功的人，呼吸差可以达到 9-18 厘米，还可以使呼吸频率减低。一般人每分钟呼吸 15-20 次，而经常练功的人，呼吸频率可以减低到每分钟 6-10 次，甚至减至 2-5 次。深而缓慢的呼吸，可以使呼吸器官获得更多的休息时间，不易疲劳，也不致因运动而出现的喘气、心慌等现象。

第二节 对消化系统的作用

道家气功炼养中，由于小腹不断地做凸、凹伸缩运动，使体内代谢加强，消耗增多这样就要求，消化器官加强功能，更好地吸取食物中的养料，以满足机体的需要。所以，练功后食欲增大，尤其是感到食物味道的甘美。练气的过程中口液（古人称“灵液”、“神水”）增加，随气沉的同时咽入腹中，即可以灌溉脏腑，润泽肢体，又可以帮助消化。练功可以促使消化器官中的腺体分泌出更多的消化液，胃肠道蠕动加强，血液循环改善，所以，食物容易被消化吸收。

丹田凸、凹的呼吸运动，使内气对胃肠、肝、脾等器官起着良好的机械按摩作用，因而也促进了这些器官的功能。

第三节 对神经器官的作用

人体的一切活动，都是在神经系统的调节下进行的。相反，各种运动，对神经系统都产生相应的影响，并促使其机能得到改善。习练道家气功，时刻要求，肢体上下相随、内外合一、心静神宁、觉明绝象。以使身体各部位与神意高度的协调统一。在这样的条件下，内气由“内景隧道”循环大、小周天、四肢百骸，提高和加强了神经系统支配运动器官的功能。经常习练不懈，神经系统的兴奋和灵活性也会得到改善，对外界刺激的反应更快、更准确，使体内各器官、系统的活动更灵活、协调、完整。同时，也提高大脑的指控功能，表现在：一能入睡快，睡的香，是治疗神经衰弱的一种有效方法；二是学习时，大脑特别清醒，效率高，质量好。经常习练道家气功，可使人体与大脑的耐受力增强，对外邪入侵的抵抗力都明显提高，所以不畏严寒酷暑，能辟外邪除疾病而长寿。

第四节　对心血管系统的作用

习练道家气功，可以保持心血管系统的健康，预防高血压和动脉血管硬化。道家气功的运动特点是螺旋式，圆形运动与气循环，丹田凸、凹紧密配合。在多方向大幅度的缠、绕、绞、转和压气、提气、沉气、发气的内外运动过程中，使动脉血管和淋巴，得到了柔和舒张，保持血管和淋巴的弹性，加强了血管循环的畅通无阻与淋巴的新陈代谢。同时交感神经的反映在练习过程中相应减弱，而副交感神经的反映相对增强。从而改变了机体的异常反映，促使血管循环正常。因此，道家气功的炼养对延缓心血管的衰老起着积极的作用。

第三章 练习气功注意事项

学习任何一项技能，都要顺其自然规律，由浅入深，由简至繁，逐步提高。在练习中必须遵守“八要”，当忌“三害”，不能太饥、太饱、胡思、愤怒。

第一节 遵守八要当忌三害

八要是：

1. 心定神宁、

2. 神宁心安、

3. 心安清静、

4. 清静无物、

5. 无物气行、

6. 气行绝象、

7. 绝象觉明、

8. 觉明则神气相通，万象归根。

三害不明者，容易走火入魔，明了才可以得到益处。三害之弊病是什麽呢？是拙力、努气、挺胸提腹。若用拙力，四肢百骸血脉不能流通，筋络不能舒畅，全身发拘，手脚也不会和顺，周身为拙力所滞，滞于何处，何处成疾病。如果练至努气，气太刚盛，容易折肺。肺为滞气所排挤，易生满闷肺炸诸症。若挺胸提腹，则气逆乱行，终不能下归丹田、两足似浮萍无根。心君不和，即万法也不能至中和之地步。所以练习时不可犯“三害”之弊病。

第二节 练习气功注意事项

练功中如果太饥饿，则没有气力。太饱容易伤脾胃，胡思乱想易误入邪途异端。忿怒则气暴，不易循行大、小周天。在练功中不可以随便谈笑、唾涎、大小便。如果随便谈笑，则精神分散而不易专心至致。唾涎则口干舌燥，水火不济，炎火上生。大小便则气易泄，力易散。

练功后，不能急于饮食、坐卧，要慢慢散步。长言说的好："功后行走百步，到老不进药铺"。

要持之以恒，习练不懈。道家气功也同其它功夫锻炼同样，贵在持久，切不可以"三天打鱼，两天晒网"，或认为功理太高、功法太难，自己笨拙学不会，或认为功夫太易，自己已经有了很高的道行了等等。练功者只有虚心求教，努力深造，才可以做到心中虚空、神态自然，精气通畅。

第三节 练功不可自专自用

练习道家气功，不可以自专自用，而固执不通，凝滞不灵。专求重者则沉重不活，专求气者则拘泥不通，专求轻者则神浮涣散。总而言之，身外形顺者，无形中自然增加气力。身内中合者，无形中自生灵气。

练习中做到，呼吸没有声音，出入要绵绵不断，若存若亡的"息息"即真息。因而，称有声为风息，虽无声不细为气息，出入滞涩是喘息。这样都不合于道家气功的要旨，因为"守风则气散，守气则息劳，守喘则气结。"所以风、气、喘三息，都不可以做到："悠、缓、细、匀、静、绵、深、长"八法，只有做到了真息的八法，才会使神态安稳，心情愉快。如果练至功行圆满之时，凝神于丹田，则身体自然重如泰山，将神气合一，化成虚空，身体自然轻似鸿羽，所以练习时不可固执一方。如果得到其中的奥秘，亦是若有若无，勿望勿助，若虚若实之意，不勉而中不思而得，从容中入道无形中而生。先师曰："精养灵根气养神，道家气功道行真。丹田练就长寿宝，万两黄金不与人。"

道家气功奥理高，
勤习默练细推敲。
功夫无息法自修，
天长日久见奇效。

第四章 炼气十八功

内气循行，点穴卸骨诸术，都以炼气养身为本。在名师传授下，收敛先天气，习练行、走、坐、卧诸功，施抱无守一之方法，循大周天、小周天、小小周天之气，达到炼性修真之目的。从妄为、有为而至于无为。

人体十二经络、奇经八脉，与五脏六腑息息相关，阴经通于脏阳经通于腑。气功大师、武术名家，治病疗疾，点穴截气，破脏腑之调节，都因明经知脉所为。

中国武当道家气功，开始练习呼吸时，吸气、舌顶上腭；呼气、舌守下腭。待气血循行通畅、顺当后，练功时舌顶上腭不变。

武当气功

第一节　无极功

无极功法合乾坤，
浑然无物顶头悬。
意在劳宫提涌泉，
虚心实腹气腾然。

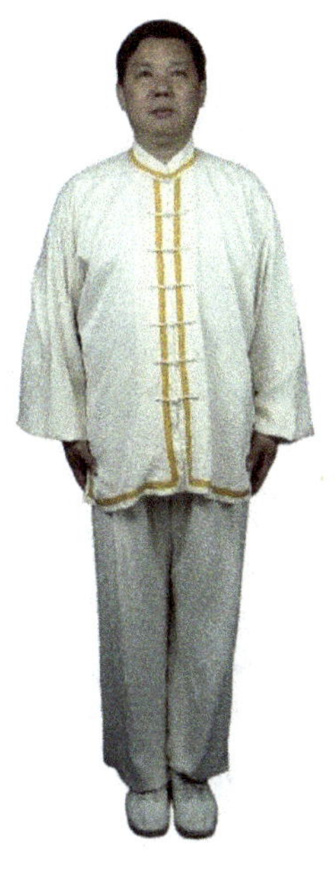

图 1-1 预备势

1）预备势

身体面南直立两脚靠拢，两臂自然下垂，食指微微上挑。目视前方，意在掌心劳宫穴（图 1-1）。

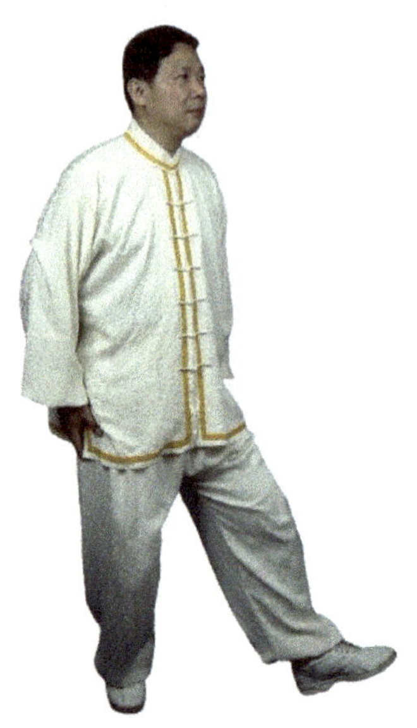

图 1-2 预备势

自然呼吸 2 次后，身体左转 45 度。左脚跟贴地面向左侧蹬出 30 厘米，脚尖内扣，脚趾抓地，脚心涌泉穴上提。目随身移，意在涌泉，气行足厥阴肝经（图 1-2）。

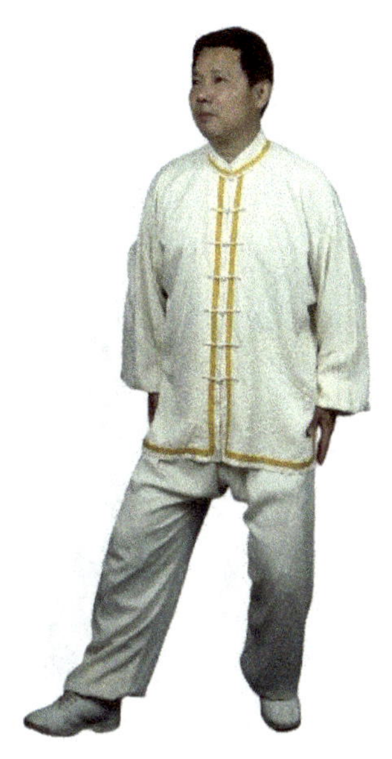

图 1-3 预备势

上动略停，重心左移，身体向右转 90 度，右脚跟贴地面向右蹬出 15 厘米，右脚尖里扣踏地。目随身移，意在玄关窍（图 1-3）。

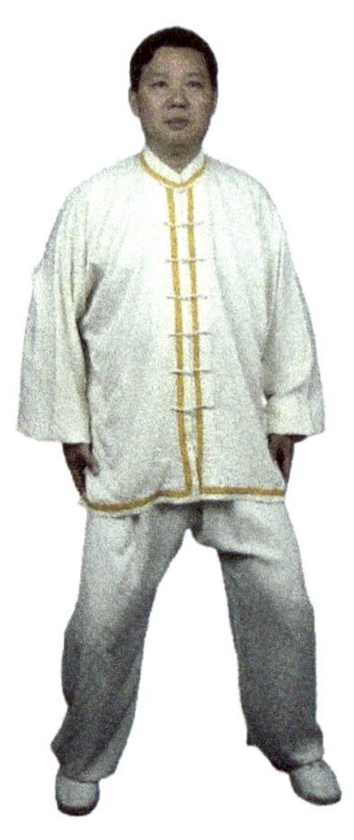

图 1-4 预备势

上动不停，体向左转 45 度，仍面向南方直立，下颌微收，头顶百会穴悬起，虚心实腹自然呼吸。目视前方，意守下丹田（图 1-4）。

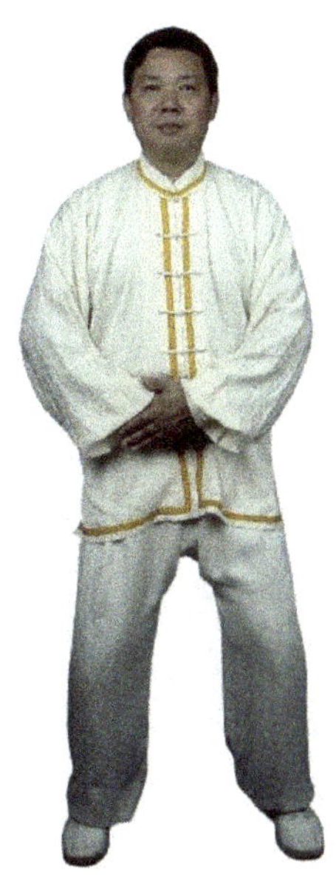

图 1-5 上提下摩

2）上提下摩

调整 2 次呼吸以后，两手由体侧向腹前划弧。掌心向内，（由于男女阴阳不同）女士右手在外，男士左手在外，两手劳宫相互叠压，轻压在下丹田上（肚脐下 4.2 厘米处亦称谓气海穴）。目微下视，意守丹田（图 1-5）。

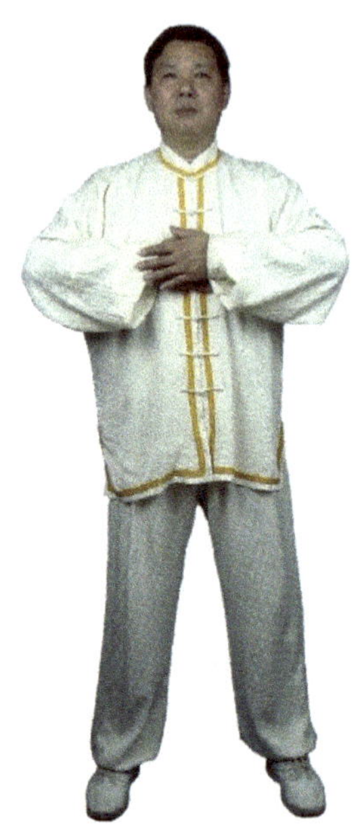

图 1-6 上提下摩

上动不停，两臂微向外旋，掌心向内贴身体向上擦行停于胸前。掌心劳宫穴与两乳之中膻中穴相对相互吸引。与之同时丹田向内凹、吸气。舌顶上腭，牙齿轻扣，目视前方，意守劳宫穴（图 1-6）。

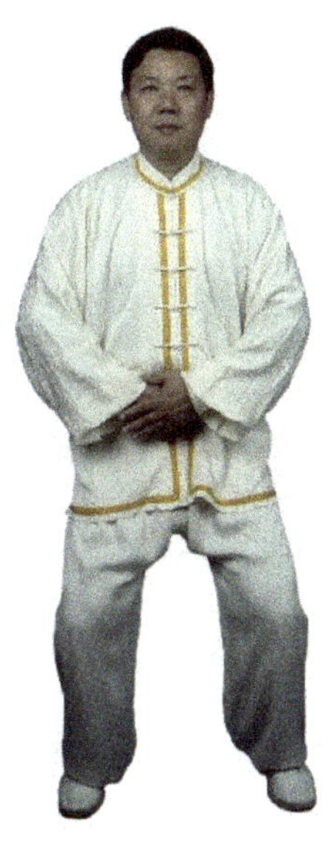

图 1-7 上提下摩

上动略停，身体重心下降，两腿屈膝下蹲成马步。同时，两臂微内旋，掌心斜向下方，贴身体向下滑动，停于脐前。与之同时，丹田向外凸起、呼气（练至气沉丹田后呼吸时舌顶上腭，不用再上下移动）。舌守下腭，牙齿微扣。目视前方，意守百会（图 1-7）。

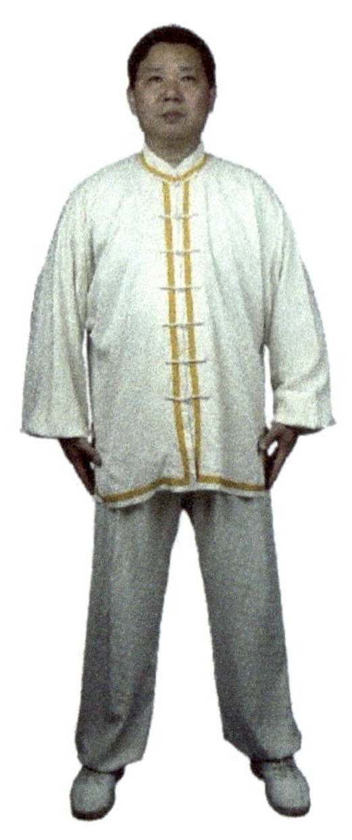

图 1-8 混元一气

3）混元一气

上动略停，调整 2 次呼吸后，两腿伸直，自然站立。同时，两手由体前分开向下划弧停于身体两侧。目视前方意守丹田（图 1-8）。

武当气功

要领与功能

无极功主要炼养丹田内气。吸气时，脚心涌泉穴、手心劳宫穴、头心百会穴，三心吸收上、中、下（阳、中、阴）3气向丹田输送。3 心之中有微凉、麻麻的感觉。呼气时由 3 心向外排气，3 心有微热的感觉（练功 100 天后热感加大）。丹田气足则水到渠成，精气往返大、小周天。初学武当道家气功，气感不太大者，可以专心意守劳宫穴一心，注重其呼吸调整。吸气抬臂时，肩要松、肘要坠。下压呼气时，脚要撑，胯要坐。会阴附近的括约肌要上提。秘决云："紧撮谷道内中提，明目辉煌顶上飞"。丹田气要意守，意念不受外界干扰。神与形相合相依，人才能以生存。无极功为内壮功修练的开始，可以使练功者，逐步达到练神还虚，复归于无极至高至上之境界。

练习方法

每次练习以 6 次或 9 次为一组，可以反复连续练习。动作的幅度大小、高低不限，以练功者的年龄老少、力量大小、体质强弱而定。

点穴

劳宫穴 PC-8[who]

涌泉穴 KC-1[who]

膻中穴 Chest Center CV-17[who]

厥阴肝经

玄关窍

百会穴 GV-20[who]

气海 CV-6[who]

第二节　推山功

推山气息聚丹田，
出纳运化不变颜。
三焦畅通气无阻，
健体护身保真元。

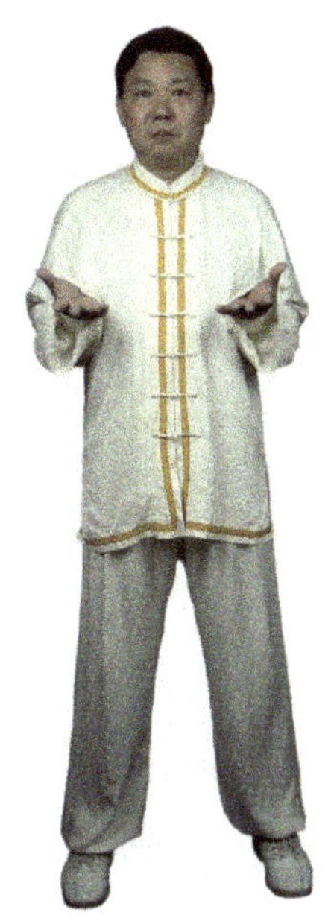

图 2-1 无极初开

1）预备势

动作方法完全同无极功预备势（参阅图 1-1、1-2、1-3、1-4）。

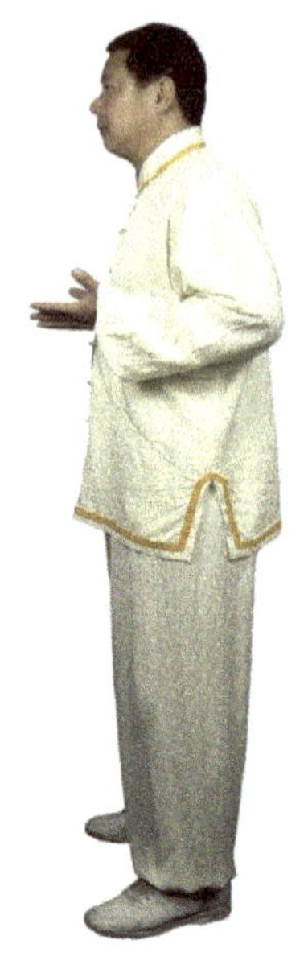

图 2-2 无极初开

2）无极初开

上动略停，调整 2 次呼吸后，两腿伸直，自然站立。同时，两臂外旋，两手随之向内上抬，掌根部停靠于两乳下。双手指尖向前，掌心向上。与之同时，丹田向内凹、吸气。舌顶上腭，牙齿轻扣，目视前方（图 2-1， 2-2）

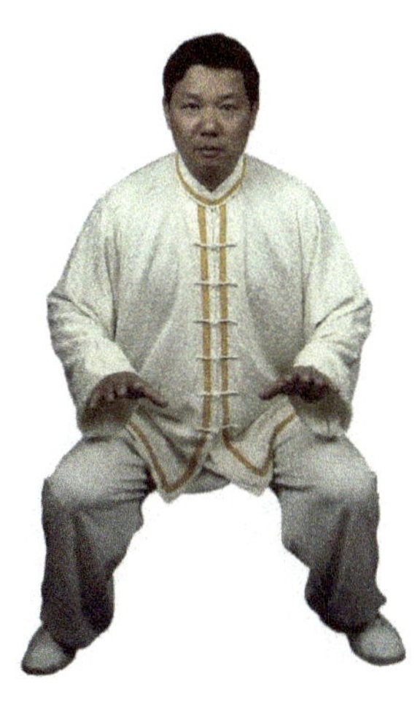

图 2-3 无极初开

上动不停，身体重心下降，两腿屈膝下蹲成马步。同时，两臂内旋，两肘合抱，手向体前弧形下按，停于腹部前面。掌心向下，指尖向前。与之同时，丹田向外凸、呼气。舌守下腭，牙齿微扣。目微下视，意在丹田，气行督任二脉（图 2-3）。

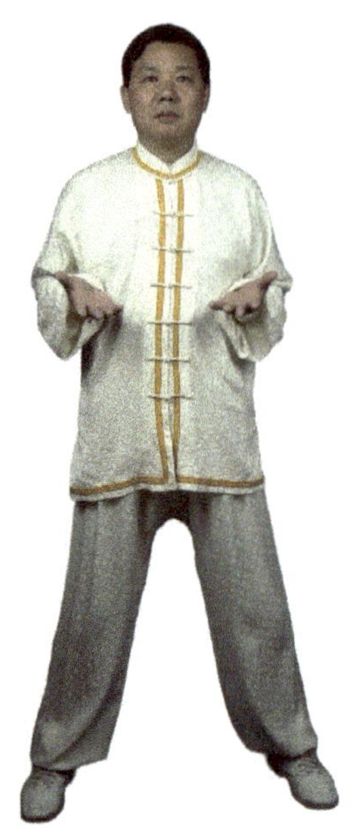

图 2-4 推山功

3）推山功

上动略停，调整 2 次呼吸后，两腿伸直 ，自然站立。同时，两臂外旋，两手随之向内上抬，掌根部停靠于两乳下。双手指尖向前，掌心向上。与之同时，丹田向内凹、吸气。舌顶上腭，牙齿轻扣，目视前方（图 2-4）。

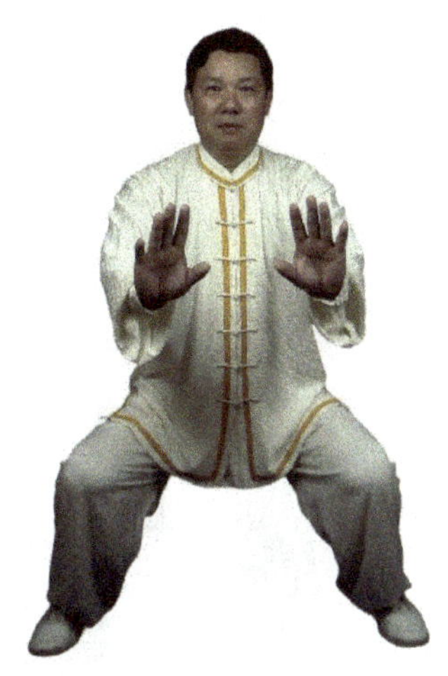

图 2-5 推山功

上动不停，身体重心下降，两腿屈膝下蹲成马步，同时，两臂内旋，掌根用力，向前平推。两掌心之间距离与两乳同宽，掌心向前，指尖向上方。与之同时，丹田向外凸、缓缓呼气。舌守下腭，牙齿微扣。目顺两掌中间向前远视，意在掌心劳宫穴（图 2-5）。

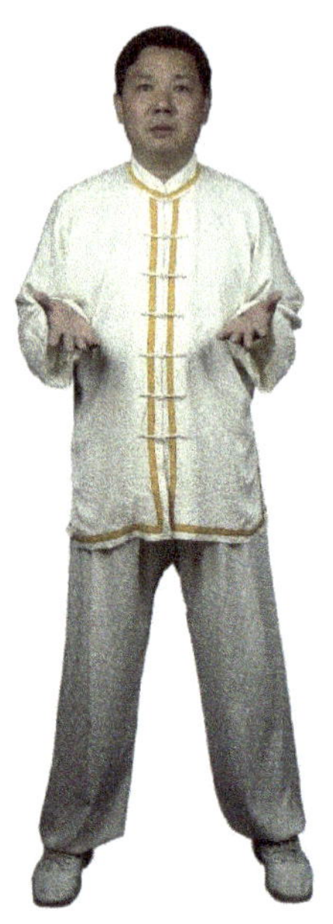

图 2-6 混元一气

4）混元一气

上动略停，调整 2 次呼吸后，两腿伸直，自然站立。同时，两臂外旋，两手随之向内上抬，掌根部停靠于两乳下。双手指尖向前，掌心向上。与之同时，丹田向内凹、吸气。舌顶上腭，牙齿轻扣，目视前方（图 2-6）。

动作方法完全同无极功混元一气（参阅图 1-8）。

武当气功

要领与功能

推山功主要练习劳宫穴向外发气。由太初无形无象的“道”生出了真元之气。真气分阴阳，阴阳衍出三才、四象、五行、八卦乃生化万物。从而重返源本，达到健体长寿之目的。抬臂呼气时，要求肩松、肘坠。动作与呼吸要紧密配合，完整一致，手停时气要吸足。精神内守，周身放松，脚趾抓地气向上行。上体正直，会阴穴与头顶心百会穴上下垂照。

呼气时，与身体下降的动作要同步，速度缓慢均匀。劳宫穴向外发气推掌时，如同推水上浮木，也好象在水中推球。周身被一种“外气”笼罩着，将混沦之气略加以收敛。用意发气，要防止太过与不及。可以采用勿望勿助之法，恰当发气行功 。用意发气，要防止太过与不及。可以采用勿望勿助之法，恰当发气行功 。

练习方法

每次练习以 6 次或 9 次为一组，可以反复连续练习。动作的幅度大小、高低不限，以练功者的年龄老少、力量大小、体质强弱而定。

点穴

真元

元气

督脉 GV[who]

任脉 CV[who]

会阴 CV-1[who]

第三节 雁飞功

大雁展翅意凌空，
鸿雁落地内丹功。
气贯双臂提双踵，
飞上落下悄无声。

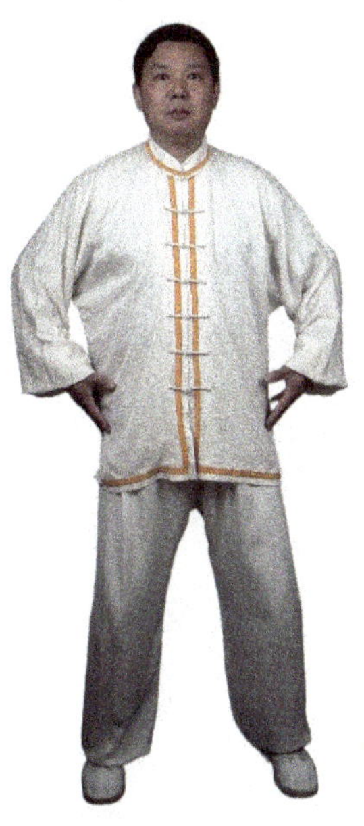

图 3-1 上下展翅

1）预备势

动作方法完全同无极功预备势（参阅图 1-1、1-2、1-3、1-4）。

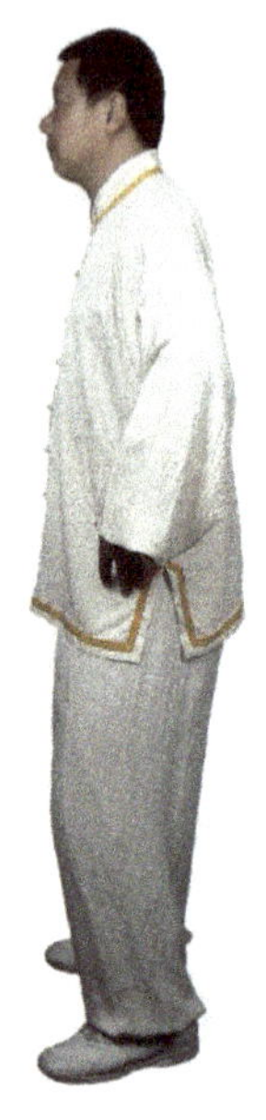

图 3-2 混元一气

2）雏燕学飞

上动不停，两手由体侧向上划弧，停于腰间，手指尖对准章门穴，掌心劳宫穴向内缩，两肘外撑，两臂屈曲似新月。肩松、肘坠。与之同时，丹田向内凹、吸气。舌顶上腭，牙齿轻扣。目向内视，意守两眼之中玄关窍（图 3-1、3-2）。

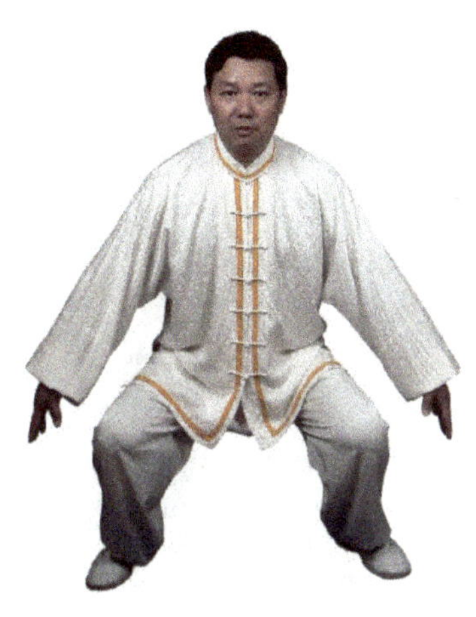

图 3-3 雏燕学飞

上动略停，身体重心下降，两腿屈膝下蹲成马步。同时，两臂内旋，双手擦脾脏、肝脏下落于腿两侧。掌心相对；指尖斜指地面（如果练功者腰背不适，双手要按摩两肾脏，向下落）。与之同时，丹田向外凸、呼气。舌守下腭，牙齿微扣，目微下视，意在阴阳上下相合（图 3-3）。

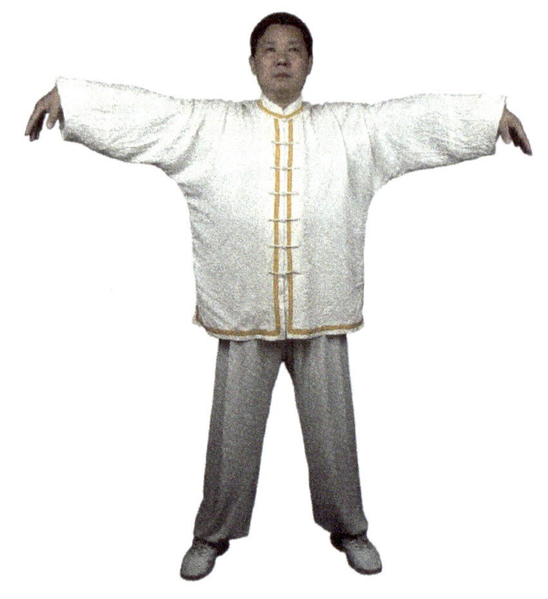

图 3-4 上下展翅

3）上下展翅

上动略停，脚跟抬起，两腿伸直，身体向上立起。同时，两手由体前向体两侧，弧形抬起，手指斜向下方，两腕关节向上用力，略高于肩。与之同时，丹田向内凹、吸气。胸开气顺，舌顶上腭，牙齿轻扣。目视前上方，意在丹田气从督脉上行至头顶心百会穴。周身一种飞上蓝天，直上金顶宫殿的感觉（图 3-4）。

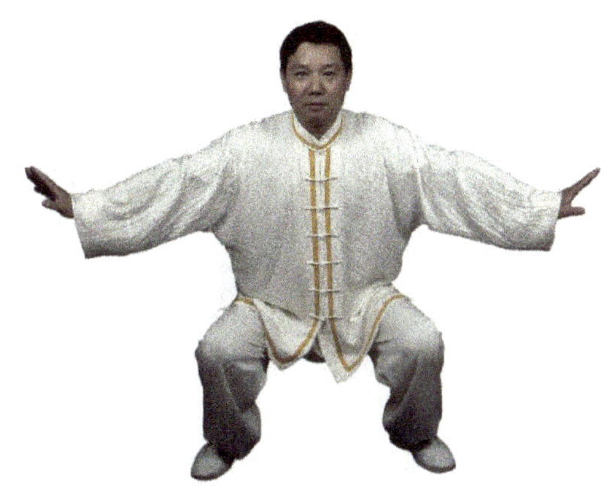

图 3-5 雏燕学飞

上动不停，身体重心下降，脚跟着地，两腿屈膝下蹲成马步。同时，腕关节下坐，两臂缓缓下落停于体两侧。指尖向外，掌心斜向下方。同时，丹田向外凸、呼气。舌守下腭，牙齿微扣。目视前方，意在肘部曲池穴下坠。周身充满了内气，象群雁落入沙滩一样舒服无比（图 3-5）。

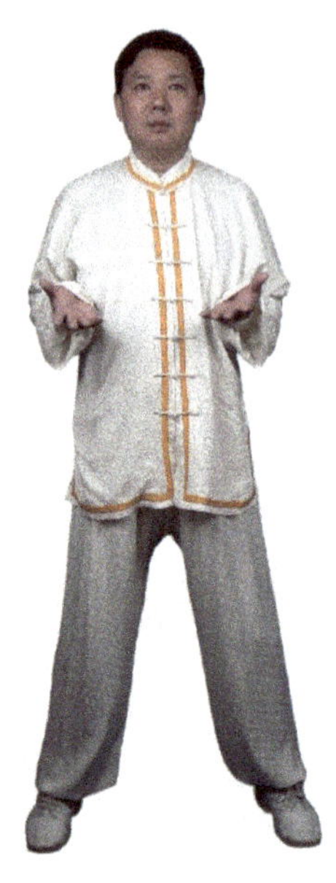

图 3-6 雏燕学飞

4）混元一气

上动略停，调整 2 次呼吸后，两腿伸直，自然站立。同时，两臂外旋，两手随之向内上抬，掌根部停靠于两乳下。双手指尖向前，掌心向上。与之同时，丹田向内凹、吸气。舌顶上腭，牙齿轻扣，目视前方（图 3-6）。

动作方法完全同无极功混元一气（参阅图 1-8）。

武当气功

要领与功能：

练习雁飞功，以起落提踵、行气为核心，是一种以呼吸为主的养生内修功夫。抬臂上飞时要求：头一直上顶与脚掌蹬地展体一致，一齐使整个身体像飞上天空一样。脚心涌泉与百会穴相照，吸气要缓慢细长，如抽丝一般，即长、匀而不断。向下落地时脚趾抓地，涌泉穴上提，身体上下连贯如一，节节相通，缓慢均匀地向下压气。肩松气则下行到肘，肘坠则气下行到腕关节，腕坐则气贯指梢。髋松则气下行到膝，膝扣则气行下落至涌泉。

行气时，要求凝神净虑，做到：轻、缓、匀、长，深。轻，呼吸轻细；缓，进气呼出缓慢；匀，呼吸节拍匀和；长，呼吸间隔时间要长；深，气渗进四肢白骸，通达周身。

练习方法：

每次练习以 6 次或 9 次为一组，可以反复连续练习。动作的幅度大小、高低不限，以练功者的年龄老少、力量大小、体质强弱而定。

点穴

章门穴 LV-13
劳宫穴 PC-8[who]
玄关窍
督脉 GV[who]
百会穴 s GV-20[who]
曲池穴 LI-11[who]
涌泉穴 KC-1[who]

第四节　鹤拗功

白鹤功练人长寿，
拗翔体如微微风。
大千世界出尘看，
心田自有灵息通。

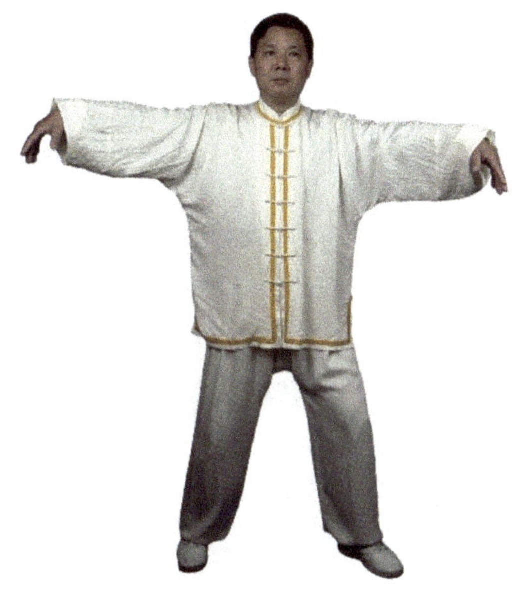

图 4-1 左拗飞

1）预备势

动作方法完全同无极功预备势（参阅图 1-1、1-2、1-3、1-4）。

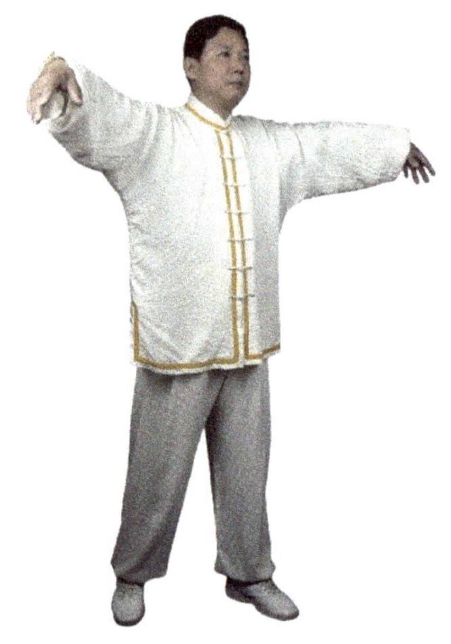

图 4-2 左拗飞

2）左拗飞

上动略停，调整 2 次呼吸后，体向左转 45 度，重心为左六、右四，右脚跟提起成左六四步。同时，身体向左上方展开，两臂随身体转动，由体侧，向左上方弧形向上缓慢飞起，肩松、肘坠，腕关节向上顶劲，略高于肩。指尖斜向下指地面，掌心向内，劳宫穴遥对足三里穴。同时，丹田向内凹、吸气。舌顶上腭，牙齿轻扣。目随身移，意在左腕部内关、外关穴（图 4-1、4-2）。

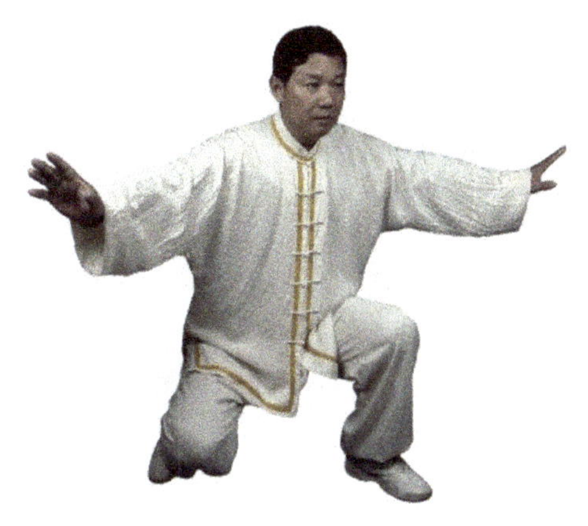

图 4-3 左拗飞

上动不停。身体重心下降，两腿屈膝下蹲成左六四步。同时，两腕关节向下屈，两臂下落停于体两侧。指尖斜向上方，掌心向下。与之同时，丹田向外凸、呼气。舌守下腭牙齿微扣。目视远方，意在中指尖中冲穴，气行手厥心阴包经（图 4-3）。

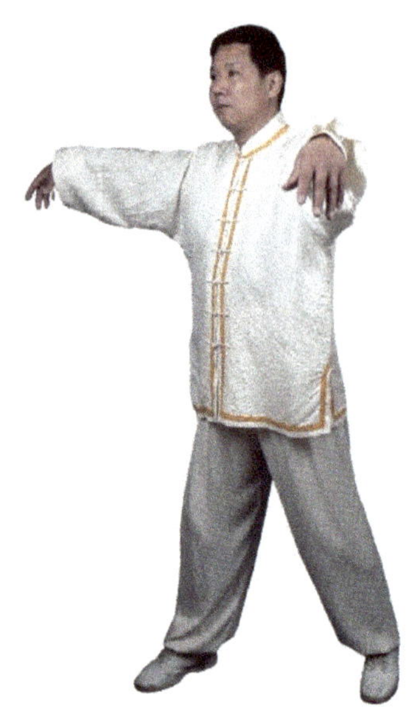

图 4-4 右拗飞

3）右拗飞

上动略停，身体向右转动 90 度，重心为右六左四，左脚跟提起成右六四步。同时，身体向右上方弧形升起，肩松，肘坠，腕关节用力上抬，略高于肩膀。手指尖斜指地面，掌心向内，劳宫穴遥对足三里穴相互挤压。同时，丹田微微内凹、吸气。舌顶上腭，牙齿轻扣。目随身移，意在右腕内关、外关穴（图 4-4）。

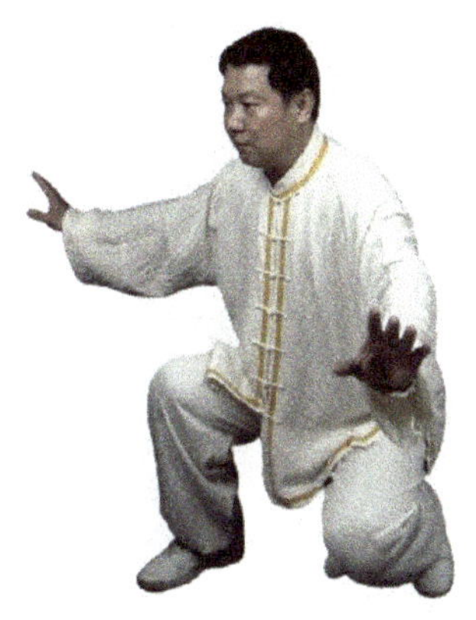

图 4-5 右拗飞

上动不停，身体重心下降，两腿屈膝下蹲成右六四步。同时，两腕关节向下坠，两臂下落斜，停于身体两侧。掌心向下，指尖斜向上方。同时，丹田向外凸、呼气。舌守下腭，牙齿微扣。目视前方，意在中指尖中冲穴，气行手厥阴心包经（图 4-5）。

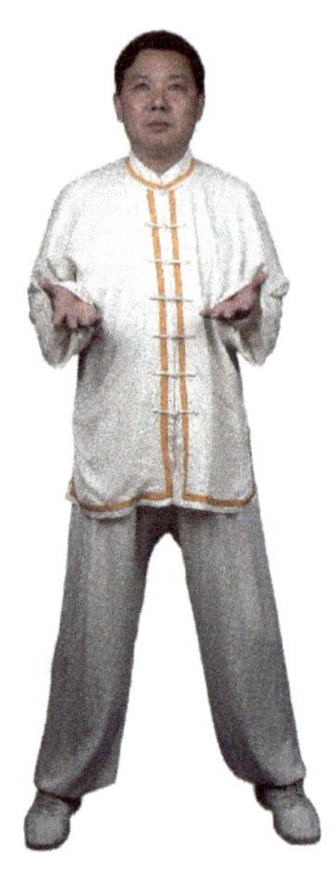

图 4-6 转身归元

4）转身归元

上动略停，身体左转 45 度。调整 2 次 呼吸后，两腿伸直，自然站立。同时，两臂向外侧旋，两手随之向内上抬，掌根部停靠于两乳下。指尖向前，掌心向上。与之同时，丹田向内凹、吸气。舌顶上腭，牙齿轻扣，目视前方（图 4-6）。

动作方法完全同无极功混元一气（参阅图 1-8）。

武当气功

要领与功能：

练习鹤拗功，整个动作必须连贯协调，体转时要以腰部为轴，身体保持中正，不可前俯后仰，左斜右外。手背要自然弯曲，手腕的上升与下降，要随动作升而用力上领，随动作降而坐腕挑指。整个动作转体上升时吸气，身体重心下降时呼气，要均匀自然，不可强求。

练功时还要注意 3 挺：脖颈自然上挺，则气贯注百会穴；挺腰舒身，则气贯注四肢；挺膝下扣，则气恬神守。

鹤拗功是以练习精、气、神为主的功法。人的生命长短，全系精、气、神之盈亏。坚持经常，持之以恒练功，可以使精足、气全、神旺。

练习方法：

每次练习以 6 次或 12 次为一组，可以反复习炼。动作的幅度、大小、高低不限，以个人年龄、力量大小、体质强弱而定。

点穴

劳宫穴 PC-8[who]

三里 ST-36

内关 PC-6[who]

外关 TB-5

中冲 PC-9[who]

厥阴心包经 PC[who]

百会穴 GV-20[who]

第五节　托天功

托天提鼎在脊端，

恍惚中间意念专。

玄祖稳坐金顶宫，

虚无里面固金丹。

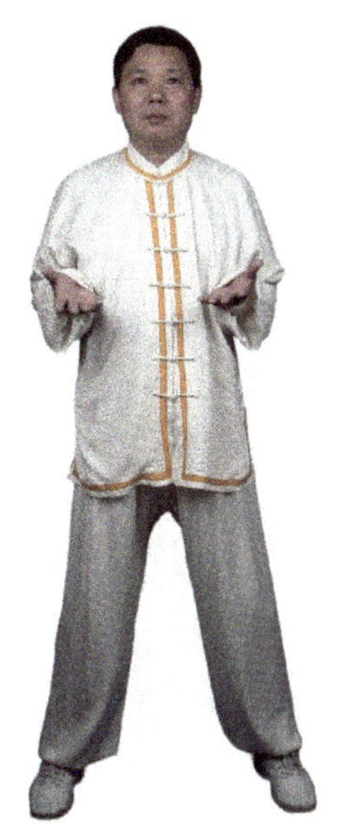

图 5-1 阴按阳托

1）预备势

动作方法完全同无极功预备势（参阅图 1-1、1-2、1-3、1-4）。

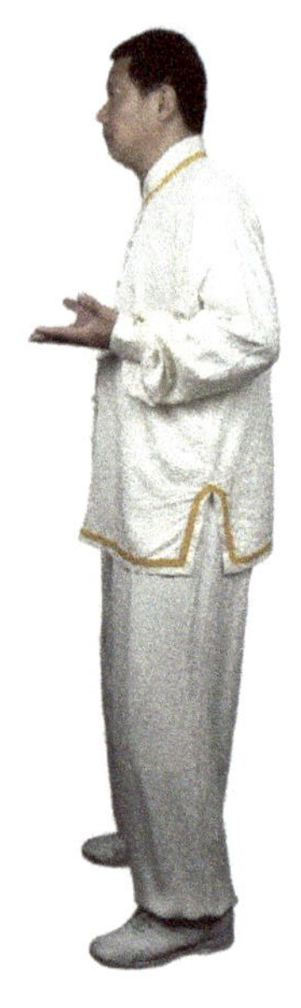

图 5-2 阴按阳托

2）阴按阳托

上动略停，调整 2 次呼吸后，两腿伸直，自然站立。同时，两臂外旋，两手随之向内上抬，掌根部停靠于两乳下。双手指尖向前，掌心向上。与之同时，丹田向内凹、吸气。舌顶上腭，牙齿轻扣，目视前方（图 5-1、5-2）。

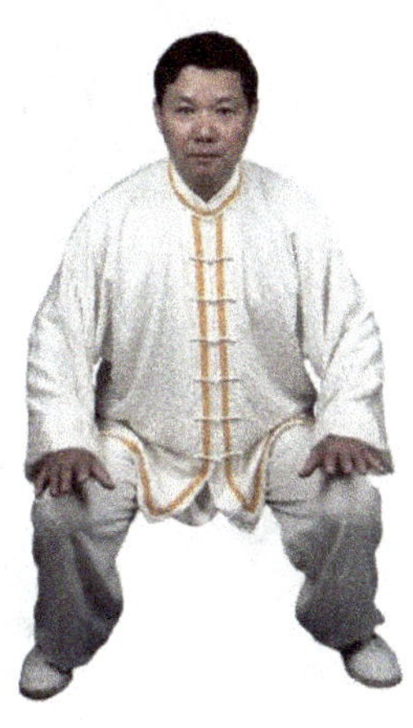

图 5-3 阴按阳托

上动不停，身体重心下降，两腿屈膝下蹲成马步。同时，两臂内旋，两肘合抱，手向体前弧形下按，停于腹前。掌心向下，指尖向前方。同时，丹田向外凸、呼气。舌守下腭，牙齿微扣。目微下视，意在丹田，气行督任二脉（图 5-3）。

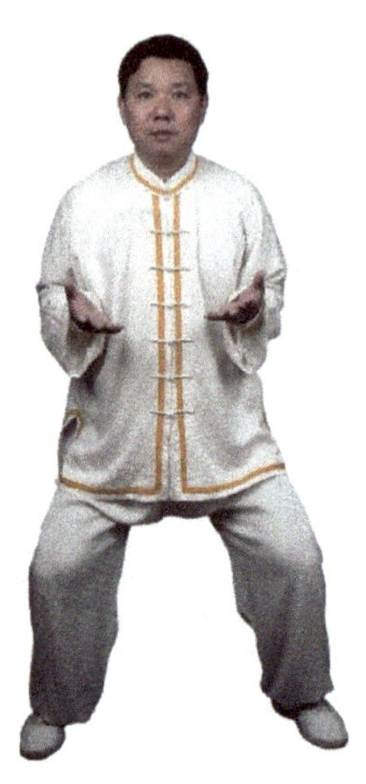

图 5-4 托天固丹

3）托天固丹

上动略停，两腿伸直，身体自然站立。两臂外旋上翻，两手随之向上划弧，掌根倚在胸前神封穴上。掌心向上，指尖斜指前上方（图 5-4）。

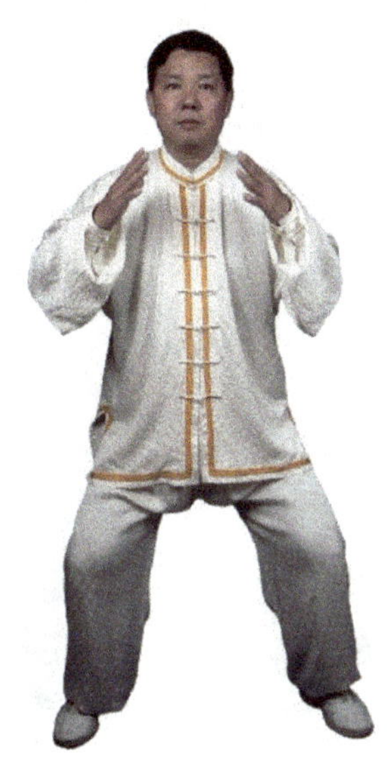

图 5-5 托天固丹

紧接上动，两腿微屈下蹲成高马步。两肘相抱相合，指尖外摆向上，两掌靠拢，掌心相对。1 段、2 段两动作的吸气，是一气吸成。丹田向内凹、缓缓吸气。舌顶上腭，牙齿轻扣。目视劳宫穴，意在玄关窍（图 5-5）。

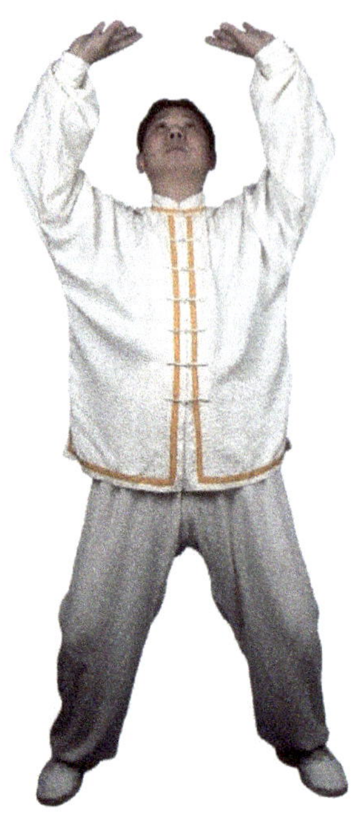

图 5-6 托天固丹

上动不停，两腿伸直，身体立起。两臂内旋上翻，两手上推成阳掌，掌心向上，指尖相对托天，停于头顶上方。与之同时，丹田向外凸、呼气。舌守下腭，牙齿微扣。身体微向后倾，目从两眼中间向上远视，意在头顶前神庭穴（图 5-6）。

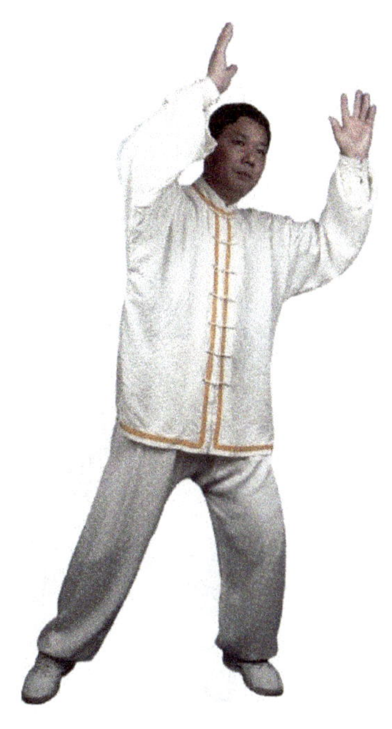

图 5-7 神龙摆尾

4）神龙摆尾

上动略停，两臂外旋，两手向下滑动，指尖向上，掌心劳宫穴相对。两手相距 30 厘米，停于额头左前上方。同时，以腰为轴带动整体向左摆动，身体重心微向下降为左六右四步（图 5-7）。

上动不停，以腰为轴带动整体向右摆动，身体重心继续向下降为右六左四步。

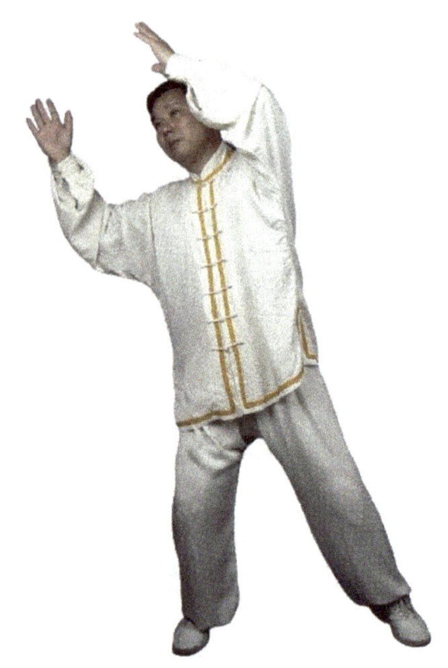

图 5-8 神龙摆尾

紧接上动，身体向左转，身体重心落于两腿之间，下蹲成马步。同时，两手由右上方向下、向左下滑动，停于胸部华盖穴两侧，指尖向前上方，小指相旁倚。与之同时，丹田向内凹、缓缓吸气，以上 3 动作一气吸成。舌顶上腭，牙齿轻扣，目随身转，意在小指少泽穴，气行手太阳小肠经（图 5-8）。

5）下按还原

动作方法完全同无极功混元一气（参阅图 1-8）。

武当气功

要领与功能：

练习托天功，神气元活贯通，形势曲折和顺，动作自然放松，周身一体随意摆动。上起托天时，身体应该保持正直，以腰为轴，两臂屈曲，两掌尽量向前上方托展。两脚不可离开地面，脚趾抓地。脚心涌泉穴上提、掌心劳宫穴上托、头顶心百会穴上悬， 3 心一齐用力向上，使内气向上发动，身体微向后仰，展腹顶肘。托天的动作要与呼气同步，一肢动百肢齐摇，一静无有不静。要求做到：和而不流，无过不及。

神龙摆尾的左摆、右摇、下蹲 3 个动作要一气吸成。吸则身动，不吸则身静。腰脊为一身之主宰，对健身壮体起着重要的作用。脊为督脉循行之途径，因而，脊背要中正放松，以帮助内气运行。随时要注意腰腹不可以前挺，这样可以使动作更加完整，扫除头重脚轻之弊经常练习托天功，有助于气通后 3 关。后三关是指督脉路线上 3 处气血不易通过的关口位置。后三关一般是指：脊椎下端尾闾关、夹脊辘轳关（华佗夹脊）、脑后玉枕关。精气由后 3 关逆督脉上至头顶百会穴；而后，下撞玄关窍沿任脉，经舌顶、下守、过膻中，直入丹田。此功法调动人体生命的潜力，以精神支配肉体，以意念控制神经，有病则除病，无病则养体，逐步达到延年益寿之目的。

练习方法：

每次练习以 6 次或 9 次为一组，可以反复连续练习。动作的幅度大小、高低不限，以练功者的年龄老少、力量大小、体质强弱而定。

武当气功

点穴

督脉 GV[who]

任脉 CV[who]

神封穴 KI-23[who]

劳宫穴 PC-8[who]

玄关窍)

神庭穴 GV-24[who]

华盖 CV-20[who]

少泽 SI-1[who]

太阳小肠经 I

涌泉穴 KC-1[who]

百会穴 GV-20[who]

尾闾关

辘轳关

玉枕 BK-9[who]

膻中

第六节　两仪功

两仪功法阴阳分，
我自忘气精神臻。
丹气有象从南转，
精气天涯向北辰。

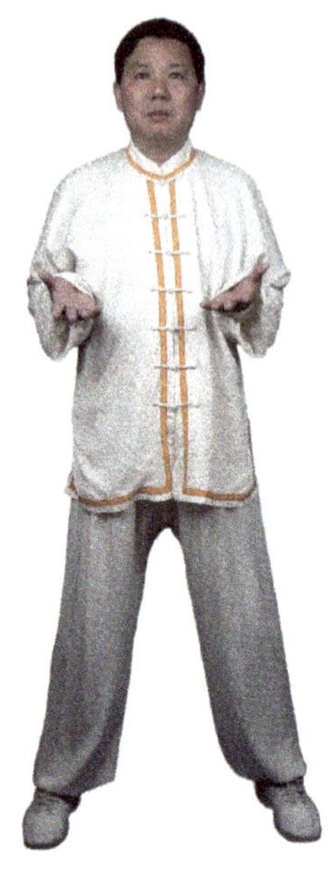

图 6-1 阴阳相合

1）预备势

动作方法完全同无极功预备势（参阅图 1-1、1-2、1-3、1-4）。

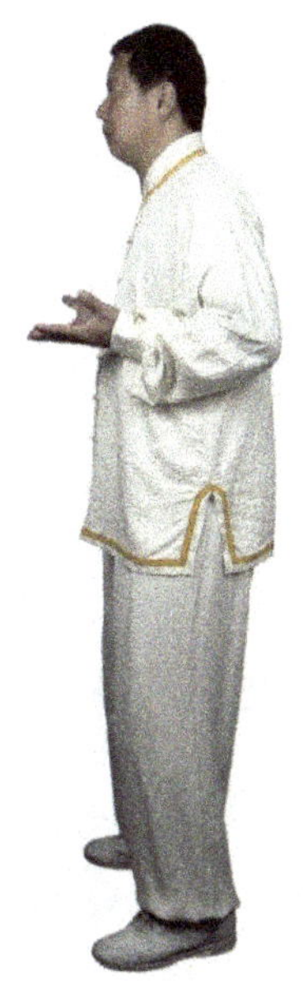

图 6-2 阴阳相合

2）阴阳相合

上动略停，调整 2 次呼吸后，两腿伸直，自然站立。同时，两臂外旋，两手随之向内上抬，掌根部停靠于两乳下。双手指尖向前，掌心向上。与之同时，丹田向内凹、吸气。舌顶上腭，牙齿轻扣，目视前方（图 6-1、6-2）。

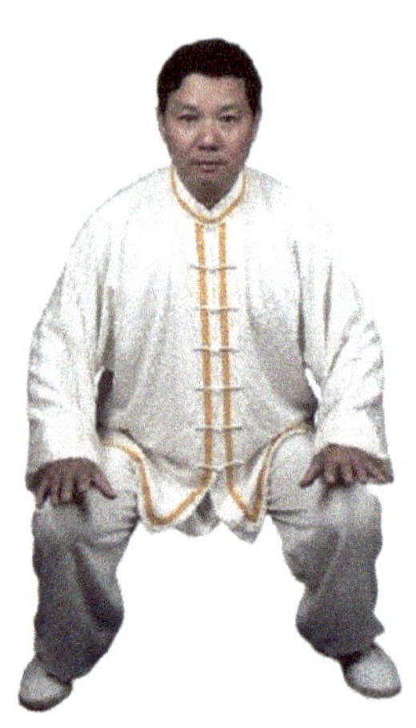

图 6-3 阴阳相合

上动不停，身体重心下降，两腿屈膝下蹲成马步。同时，两臂内旋，两肘合抱，手向体前弧形下按，停于腹前。掌心向下，指尖向前方。同时，丹田向外凸、呼气。舌守下腭，牙齿微扣。目微下视，意在丹田，气行督任二脉（图 6-3）。

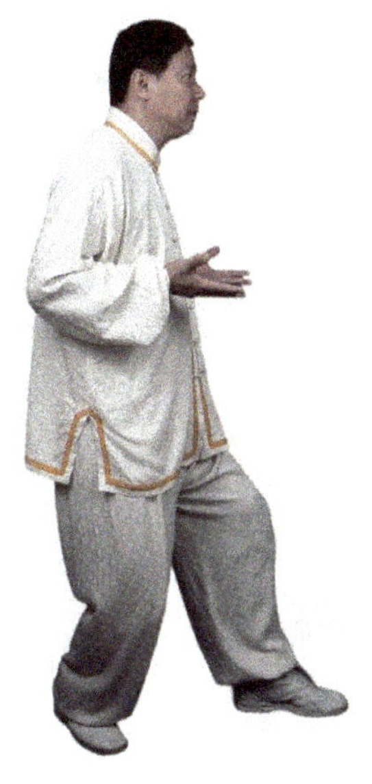

图 6-4 两仪左势

3）两仪左势

上动略停，身体重心右移。身体向左转 90 度成左六四步。左脚尖翘起，脚跟着地微向回拉。同时，两臂外旋两手由腹前向上方弧形提撩。指尖向前，掌心向上停于胸下期门穴处。与之同时，丹田向内凹、吸气。舌顶上腭，牙齿轻扣。目随身移，意在脚心涌泉穴向上提气（图 6-4）。

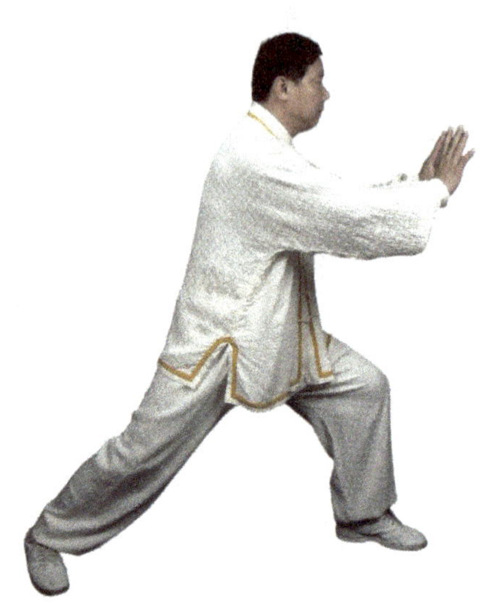

图 6-5 两仪左势

上动略停，左脚向前滑出半步，前脚掌下压，脚趾抓地。身体重心前移，左腿膝部微向下屈：右腿伸直前蹬成左弓步。同时，两臂外旋，两手由胸下向前上方弧形推出。指尖向前上方，掌心向前下方，略高于肩。与之同时，丹田向外凸、呼气。舌守下腭，牙齿微扣。目从两手拇指间远视，意在掌心劳宫穴，气行手太阴肺经（图 6-5）。

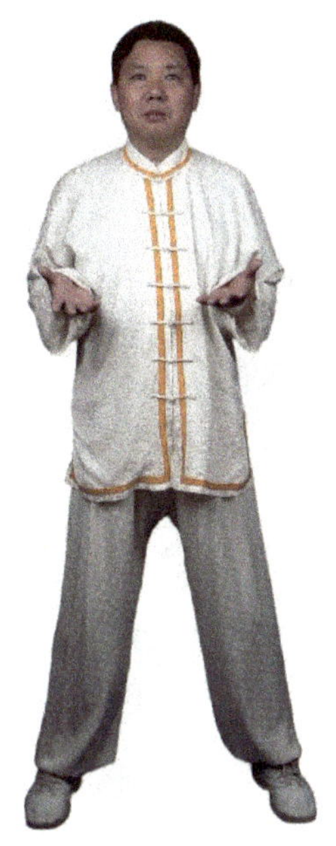

图 6-6 右转小收

4）右转小收

上动略停，身体右转 90 度。调整 2 次呼吸后，两腿伸直，自然站立。同时，两臂外旋，两手随之向内上抬，掌根部停靠于两乳下。指尖向前，掌心向上。与之同时，丹田向内凹、吸气。舌顶上腭，牙齿轻扣，目视前方（图 6-6）。

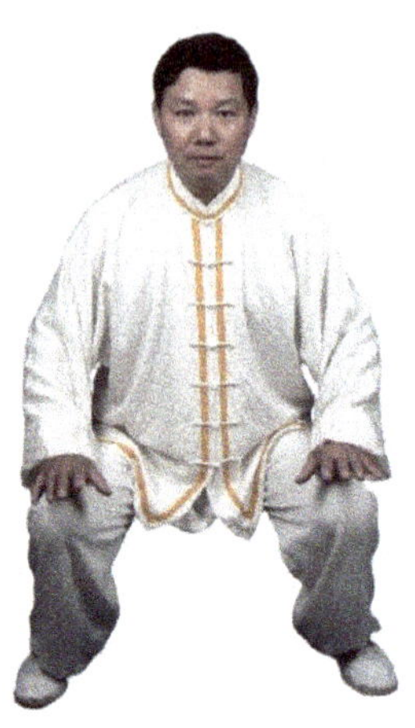

图 6-7 右转小收

上动不停，身体重心下降，两腿屈膝下蹲成马步。同时，两臂内旋，两肘合抱，手向体前弧形下按，停于腹前。掌心向下，指尖向前方。同时，丹田向外凸、呼气。舌守下腭，牙齿微扣。目微下视，意在丹田，气行督任二脉（图 6-7）。

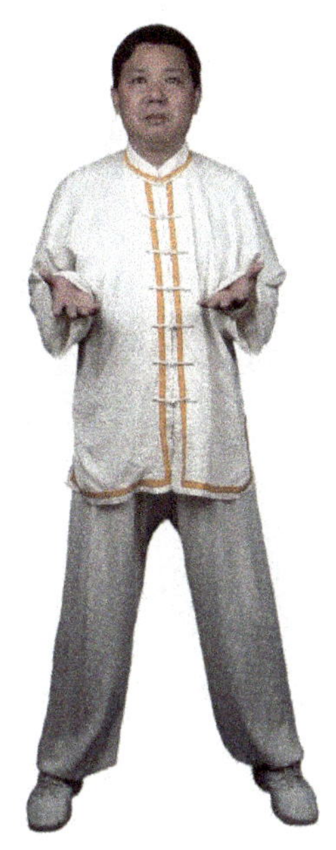

图 6-8 还原收势

5）两仪右势

动作方法完全同两仪左势，惟左右方向相反（参阅图 6-4、6-5）。

6）还原收势

上动略停，身体左转 90 度。调整 2 次呼吸后，两腿伸直，自然站立。同时，两臂外旋，两手随之向内上抬，掌根部停靠于两乳下。指尖向前，掌心向上。与之同时，丹田向内凹、吸气。舌顶上腭，牙齿轻扣，目视前方（图 6-8）。

动作方法完全同无极功混元一气（参阅图 1-8）。

武当气功

要领与功能：

两仪功法就是太极化生两仪之象。阴阳起落，动静往来，动作简，而内气腾然。当吸气时，足 3 阴之气脉与外气相互调引，循经络上行，水火相济，阴阳调合，则百病可以清除。练功吸气时，内气从丹田开始经会阴、上下鹊桥、尾闾关、腰阳关、命门穴。练功呼气时，内气经阴交诸穴下至气海穴，循行小小周天。而后，行功有一些基础时，再练习小周天、大周天功夫，则易一通百通走入正道。

两手向下按、屈前腿、登后腿动作，要与呼气配合整齐一致。意念感到一股热流，似车轮一样在小小周天运行不息。

两仪功外形的姿势要做到正确，体内的意和气才可以运行通畅，而外形、气力才可以顺当。练功时还必须做到：肩与髋、肘与膝、手与足、心与意、意与气、气与力，内外 6 合。

外 3 合要求动作圆贯协调，左右上下前后配合得当，姿势舒展大方；内 3 合就是要用心意调动气与力的运行，意到何处，内气也要运行的何处，并和劲力同至。外形随之而动，达到心神合一之境界。体质逐渐就会得到增强，转衰弱为强壮，化未老先衰为青春常在。

练习方法：

每次练习以 6 次或 12 次为一组，可以反复习炼。动作的幅度、大小、高低不限，以个人年龄、力量大小、体质强弱而定。

武当气功

点穴

督脉 GV[who]

任脉 CV[who]

期门 LV-14

涌泉穴 KC-1[who]

劳宫穴 PC-8[who]

手太阴肺经 LU[who]

会阴 CV-1[who]

鹊桥

尾闾关

腰阳关 GV-3[who]

命门穴 GV-4[who]

阴交 CV-7[who]

气海 CV-6[who]

第七节 四象功

阴阳两仪四象生，
炼神还虚理自醒。
要知药火功夫处，
气足神全丹道成。

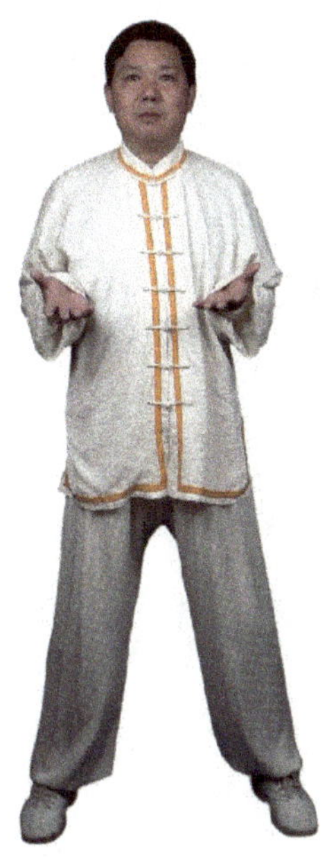

图 7-1 上提下压

1）预备势

动作方法完全同无极功预备势（参阅图 1-1、1-2、1-3、1-4）。

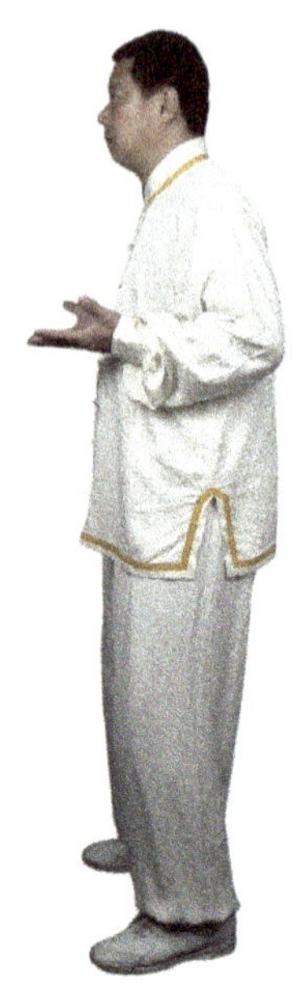

图 7-2 上提下压

2）上提下压

上动略停，调整 2 次呼吸后，两腿伸直，自然站立。同时，两臂外旋，两手随之向内上抬，掌根部停靠于两乳下。双手指尖向前，掌心向上。与之同时，丹田向内凹、吸气。舌顶上腭，牙齿轻扣，目视前方（图 7-1、7-2）。

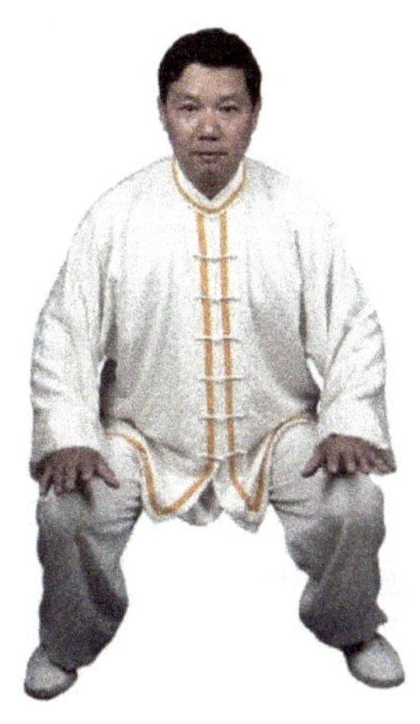

图 7-3 上提下压

上动不停，身体重心下降，两腿屈膝下蹲成马步。同时，两臂内旋，两肘合抱，手向体前弧形下按，停于腹前。掌心向下，指尖向前方。同时，丹田向外凸、呼气。舌守下腭，牙齿微扣。目微下视，意在丹田，气行督任二脉（图 7-3）。

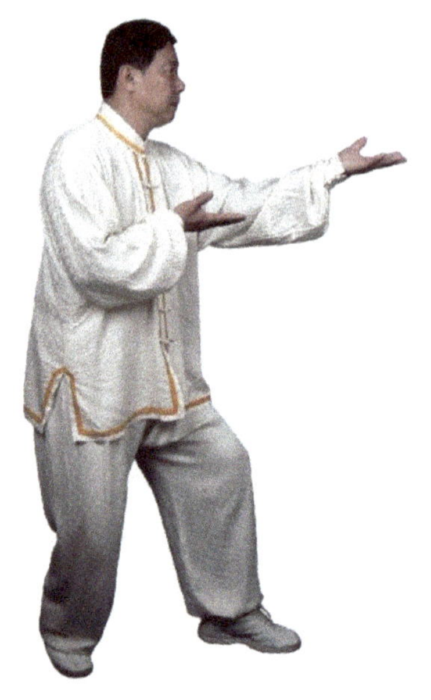

图 7-4 四象左势

3）四象左势

上动略停，身体重心微向右移动，体向左转 90 度，左脚跟离地回拉停于右脚弓前成左高虚步。与之同时，两臂外旋，双手由腹前向左上方弧形托起。左手在前于肩同高，指尖向前上方，掌心向上；右手停于左肘关节内侧，指尖向前，掌心向上。托掌同时，丹田向内凹、吸气。舌顶上腭，牙齿轻扣。目随身转，意在食指、拇指对撑（图 7-4）。

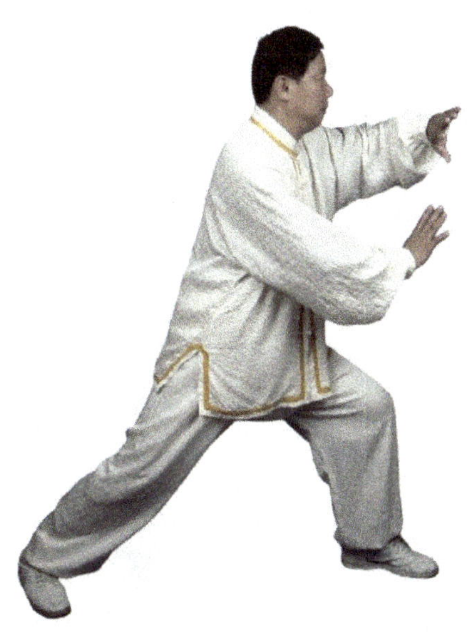

图 7-5 四象左势

上动不停，左脚向前上半步，脚尖内扣，左腿屈膝下蹲；右腿挺膝伸直成左弓步。与之同时，以腰带动双掌，臂内旋，双手在胸前转一立圆，而后，再向左上方横翻推出。左手指尖向右，掌心向前与肩同高；右手停于左掌下 10 厘米处，指尖向上，掌心向前。与之同时，丹田向外凸、呼气。舌守下腭，牙齿微扣。目视左前方，意在掌心劳宫穴（图 7-5）。

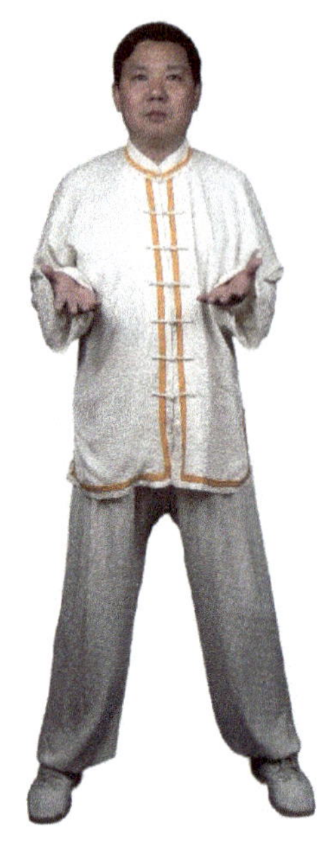

图 7-6 右转小收

4）右转小收

上动略停，身体右转 90 度。调整 2 次呼吸后，两腿伸直，自然站立。同时，两臂外旋，两手随之向内上抬，掌根部停靠于两乳下。指尖向前，掌心向上。与之同时，丹田向内凹、吸气。舌顶上腭，牙齿轻扣，目视前方（图 7-6）。

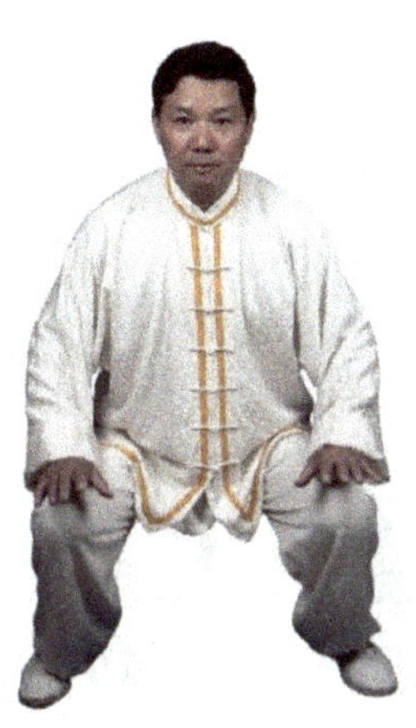

图 7-7 右转小收

上动不停，身体重心下降，两腿屈膝下蹲成马步。同时，两臂内旋，两肘合抱，手向体前弧形下按，停于腹前。掌心向下，指尖向前方。同时，丹田向外凸、呼气。舌守下腭，牙齿微扣。目微下视，意在丹田，气行督任二脉（图 7-7）。

5）四象右势

动作方法完全同四象左势，惟左右方向相反（参阅图 7-4、7-5）。

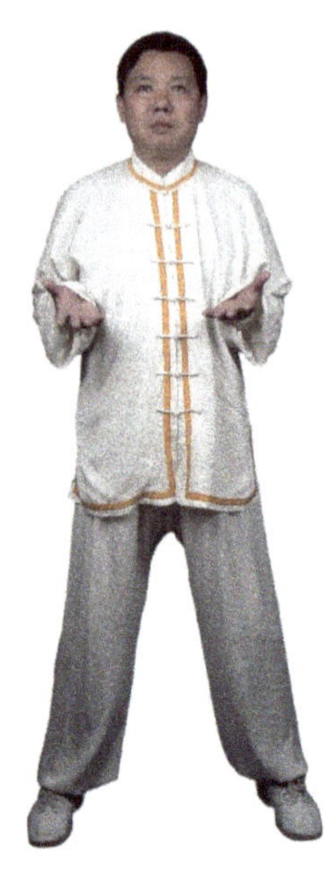

图 7-8 还原收势

6）还原收势

上动略停，身体左转 90 度。调整 2 次呼吸后，两腿伸直，自然站立。同时，两臂外旋，两手随之向内上抬，掌根部停靠于两乳下。指尖向前，掌心向上。与之同时，丹田向内凹、吸气。舌顶上腭，牙齿轻扣，目视前方（图 7-8）。

动作方法完全同无极功混元一气（参阅图 1-8）。

武当气功

要领与功能：

练习四象功时要注重“虚领顶劲，气沉丹田”的要领。这也是练习任何气功、内功，功夫者开宗明义的第一大要求。没有虚领顶劲，气则不易下沉到丹田。练习中国道家-武当气功，以养气为主，养气形势，就是要意、气、行经。气循腰间，为冲督之表现，肾气充盈，则内气运行周身，无所不至。动中求静，静中生动，动静相生，则内气因势而变异，运用无穷。左旋右转，升起降落，前进后退，都是帮助练功者内气通顺，内劲运行之形势。

练习四象功还要做到：认真细心，内外如一。周身的动作与呼吸要配合一致。注意：3 心要並、3 意要连、五行要顺达。心中安逸自然，毫无惶惶努气之感。3 心要並是指顶心百会穴往下吸上气（即阳气），脚心涌泉穴往上吸下气（即阴气），手心劳宫穴回缩吸中气。如此则上边之气易降，下边之气易升，中气也易于收回于是便能全归于一，缩于秘，集于丹田。3 意连，就是心意、气意、力意三者连贯为一个整体。

五行要顺达，是指外形进、退、顾、盼、定的动静变化要与体内心、肝、脾、肺、肾，的五脏之气互相随顺，内动外随。息调、神凝、气聚，经络之气流行畅通，循环无端，气血可以流行全身，川流不息，百脉流通，内外兼修，身心健康。

武当气功

练习方法：

每次练习以 6 次或 9 次为一组，可以反复习炼。动作的幅度、大小、高低不限，以个人年龄、力量大小、体质强弱而定。

点穴

督脉 GV[who]
任脉 CV[who]
冲脉 PV
百会穴 GV-20[who]
涌泉穴 KC-1[who]
劳宫穴 PC-8[who]

第八节 棚捋功

棚捋功法正而奇，
升清降浊调呼吸。
刚柔相济气通天，
浪峰涛山只等闲。

武当气功

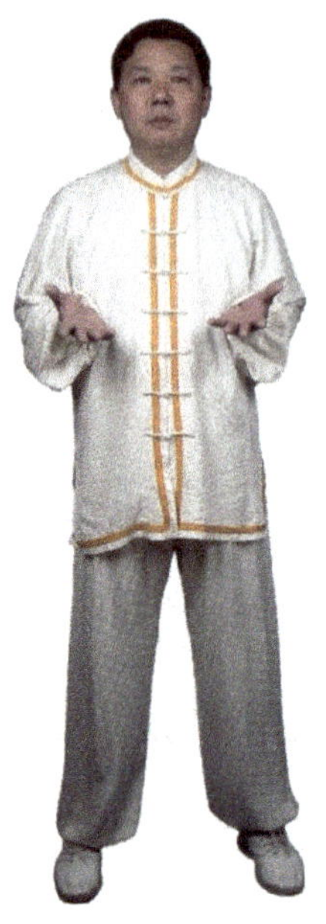

图 8-1 升清降浊

1）预备势

动作方法完全同无极功预备势（参阅图 1-1、1-2、1-3、1-4）。

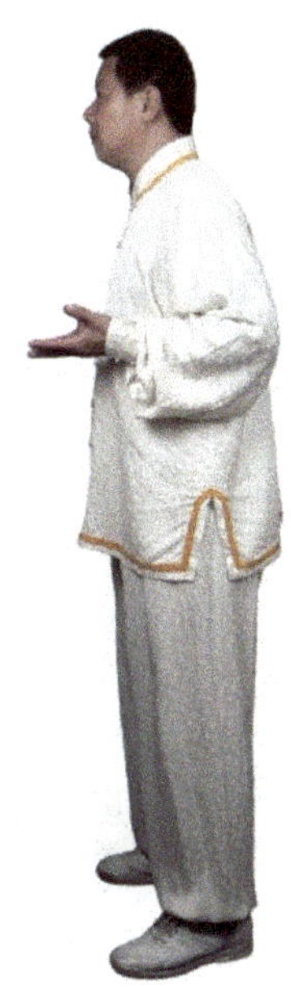

图 8-2 升清降浊

2）升清降浊

上动略停，调整 2 次呼吸后，两腿伸直，自然站立。同时，两臂外旋，两手随之向内上抬，掌根部停靠于两乳下。双手指尖向前，掌心向上。与之同时，丹田向内凹、吸气。舌顶上腭，牙齿轻扣，目视前方（图 8-1、8-2）。

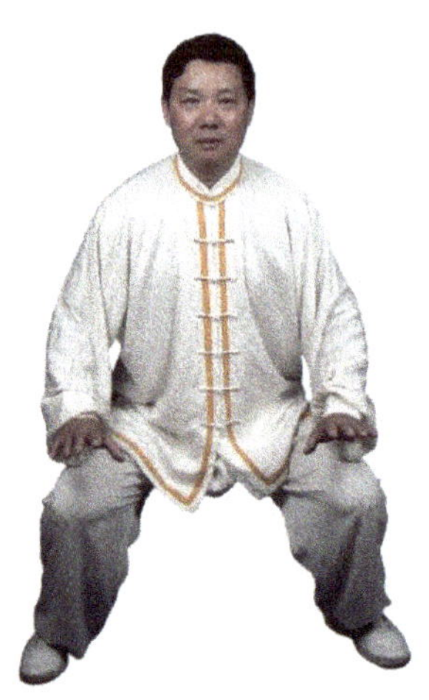

图 8-3 升清降浊

上动不停，身体重心下降，两腿屈膝下蹲成马步。同时，两臂内旋，两肘合抱，手向体前弧形下按，停于腹前。掌心向下，指尖向前方。同时，丹田向外凸、呼气。舌守下腭，牙齿微扣。目微下视，意在丹田，气行督任二脉（图 8-3）。

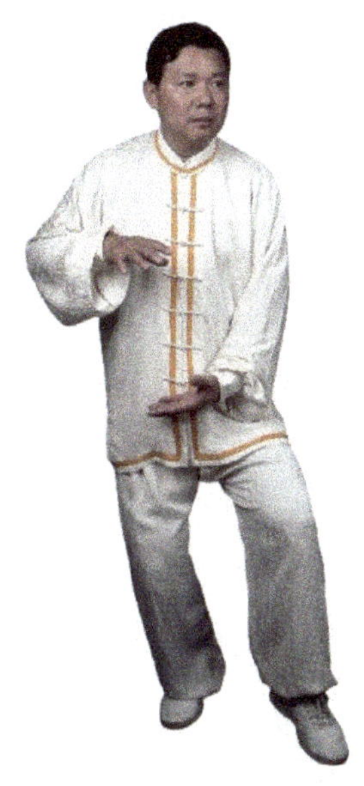

图 8-4 左棚右捋

3）左棚右捋

上动不停，身体重心升起，体向左转动 45 度自然站立。左臂歪旋，左手于左腹前翻转，掌心向上，指尖向右；右手上抬停于左胸前，指尖向左，掌心向下。两手劳宫穴相对，互相吸引。与之同时，丹田向内凹、吸气。舌顶上腭，牙齿轻扣。目微下视，意在掌心劳宫穴（图 8-4）。

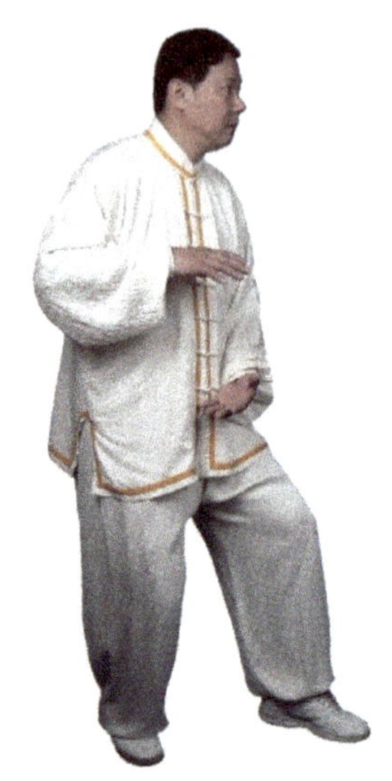

图 8-5 左棚右捋

上动略停，身体重心右移，体继续左转 45 度，左脚尖翘起，右脚跟着地成左高虚步。与之同时，两手体前抱球随之而动（图 8-5）。

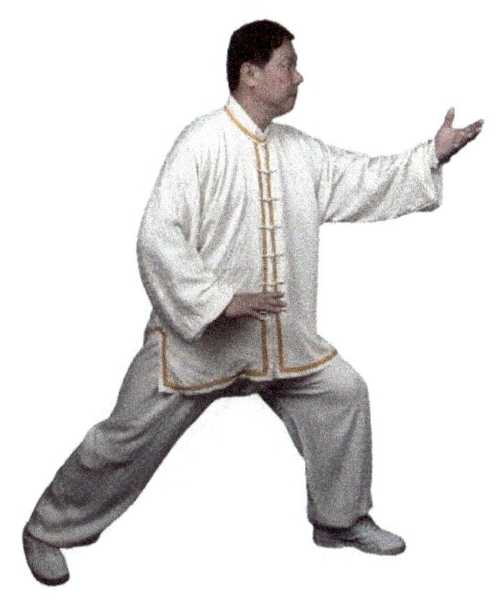

图 8-6 左棚右捋

紧接上动不停，左脚微向前移，全脚掌着地，涌泉穴上提，左腿屈膝半蹲；右腿挺膝伸直成左弓步。同时，左掌从腹前抬起，以食指领气弧形向左前上方棚出，与肩同高。食指尖向左前方，掌心向上，气行手阳明大肠经；右手从胸前向右下方斜捋，停于腹右侧水道穴旁边，气行足阳明胃经。同时，丹田向外凸、呼气。舌守下腭，牙齿微扣。目视左前方，意在双手食指商阳穴，两手分拉如抽丝一般（图 8-6）。

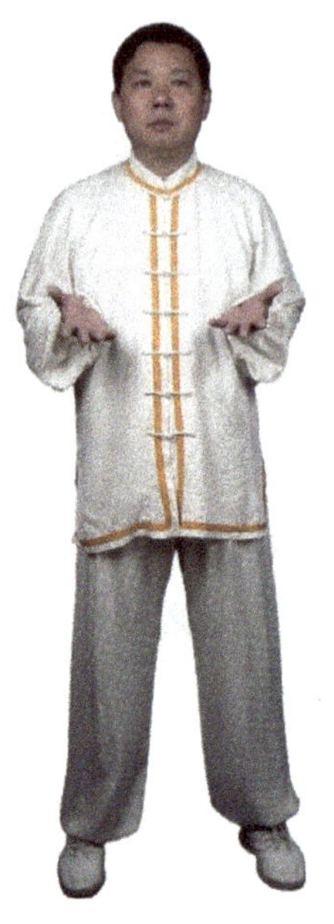

图 8-7 右转合气

4）右转合气

上动略停，身体右转 90 度。调整 2 次呼吸后，两腿伸直，自然站立。同时，两臂外旋，两手随之向内上抬，掌根部停靠于两乳下。指尖向前，掌心向上。与之同时，丹田向内凹、吸气。舌顶上腭，牙齿轻扣，目视前方（图 8-7）。

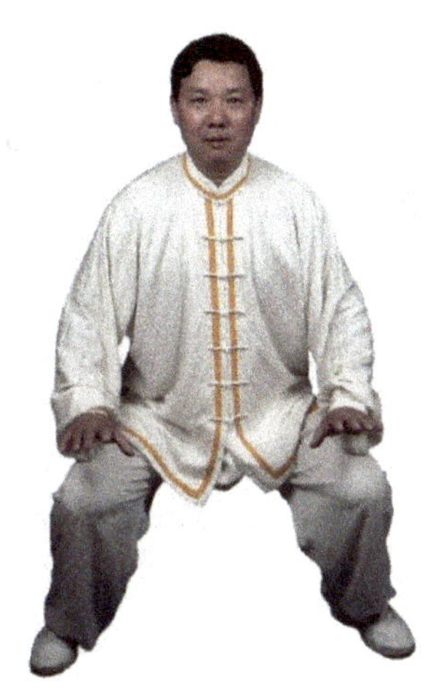

图 8-8 右转合气

上动不停，身体重心下降，两腿屈膝下蹲成马步。同时，两臂内旋，两肘合抱，手向体前弧形下按，停于腹前。掌心向下，指尖向前方。同时，丹田向外凸、呼气。舌守下腭，牙齿微扣。目微下视，意在丹田，气行督任二脉（图 8-8）。

5）右棚左捋

动作方法完全同左棚右捋，惟左右方向相反（参阅图 8-4、8-5、8-6）。

6）回身收势

动作方法完全同推山功无极初开（参阅图 2-1）。上动不停，动作方法完全同无极功混元一气（参阅图 1-8）。

武当气功

要领与功能：

练功时要注意“棚、捋”时内气的运行轨迹、经络。先由意动，以意领气，循行带脉往复冲脉上下，使气血流通。此动作大开大合，上阳下阴。两手腹前抱球后，食指相扯相拉。“棚”出时肩松、肘坠、顶腕、圆臂，5 指自然分开，食指外挑，其余 4 指微向内扣，掌心要含，气贯食指尖。“捋”下时，腕关节要塌坐，食指仍上挑，其余 4 指下抓好象在水中抓葫芦一样，整个动作不即不离，和而不流。

吸气时尽量做到没有声音，绵绵不断，无形无象，不可以滞涩喘气。人以气为本，以心为根，以息为主。天不能无阴阳，人不能无呼吸。

一呼百脉皆开，一吸百脉皆合。天地要阴阳，真气之运行，都离不开呼吸二字。练功时，呼吸一定要任其自然，合于练功之规矩。调气之法就是“轻出缓入”，呼吸用鼻为主。用以力活气顺、虚心实腹时，自然练至化境。

练习方法：

每次练习以 6 次或 12 次为一组，可以反复习炼。动作的幅度、大小、高低不限，以个人年龄、力量大小、体质强弱而定。

武当气功

点穴

督脉 GV[who]

任脉 CV[who]

劳宫穴 PC-8[who]

涌泉穴 KC-1[who]

手阳明大肠经 LI[who]

水道穴 ST-28[who]

足阳明胃经 [who]

商阳穴 LI-1[who]

带脉 GIV, GB-26[who]

冲脉 PV

第九节 琵琶功

三弹琵琶分两边，
阴阳变化理自然。
意气君来骨肉臣，
天精地灵补元丹。

武当气功

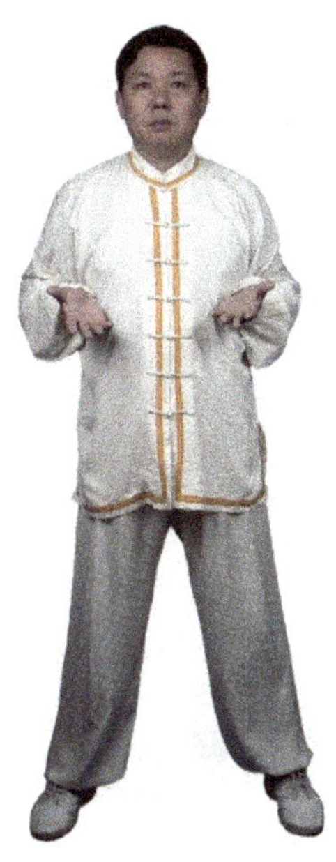

图 9-1 上下调气

1）预备势

动作方法完全同无极功预备势（参阅图 1-1、1-2、1-3、1-4）。

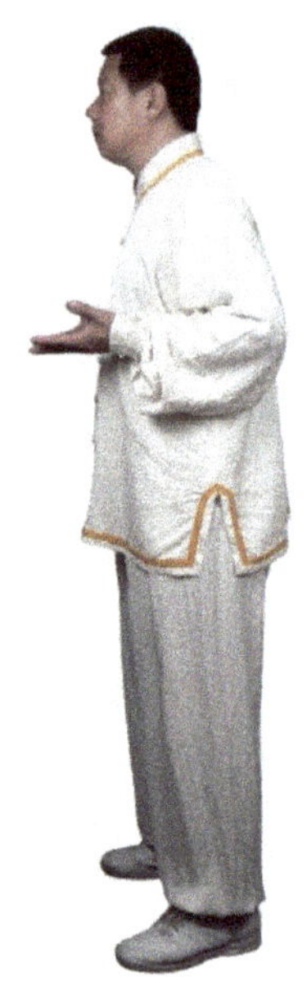

图 9-2 上下调气

2）上下调气

上动略停，调整 2 次呼吸后，两腿伸直，自然站立。同时，两臂外旋，两手随之向内上抬，掌根部停靠于两乳下。双手指尖向前，掌心向上。与之同时，丹田向内凹、吸气。舌顶上腭，牙齿轻扣，目视前方（图 9-1、9-2）。

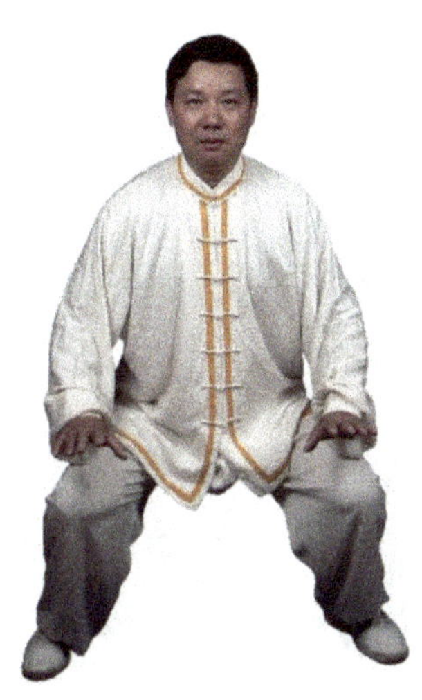

图 9-3 上下调气

上动不停，身体重心下降，两腿屈膝下蹲成马步。同时，两臂内旋，两肘合抱，手向体前弧形下按，停于腹前。掌心向下，指尖向前方。同时，丹田向外凸、呼气。舌守下腭，牙齿微扣。目微下视，意在丹田，气行督任二脉（图 9-3）。

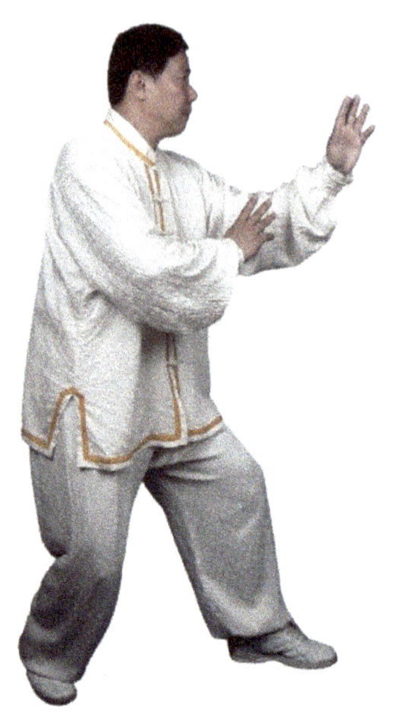

图 9-4 琵琶左势

3）琵琶左势

上动略停，身体重心右移，体向左转动 90 度，左脚尖翘起成左高虚步。同时，双手立掌向左上方钻出。左掌略高于肩，指尖向前，掌心向右；右掌停于左肘关节内侧，指尖向上，掌心向左。与之同时，丹田向内凹、吸气。舌顶上腭，牙齿轻扣。目随左手指移动，意在头顶百会穴（图 9-4）。

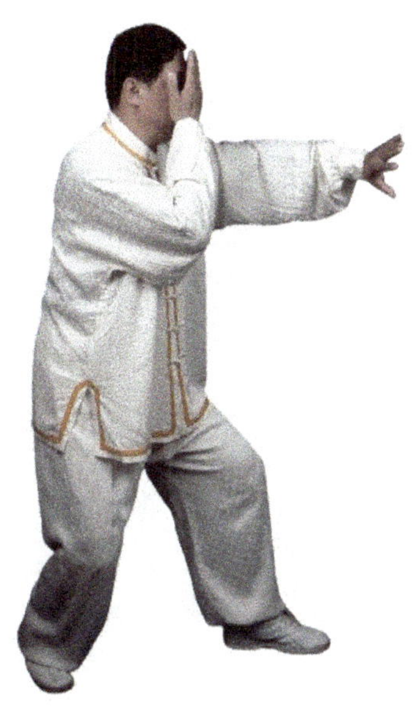

图 9-5 琵琶左势

上动不停，体微向左转，左臂外旋，左掌回拨，指尖向上，掌心劳宫穴向面部左侧四白穴；右臂内旋，右掌指用力向外弹拨，指尖向左，掌心向前（图 9-5）。

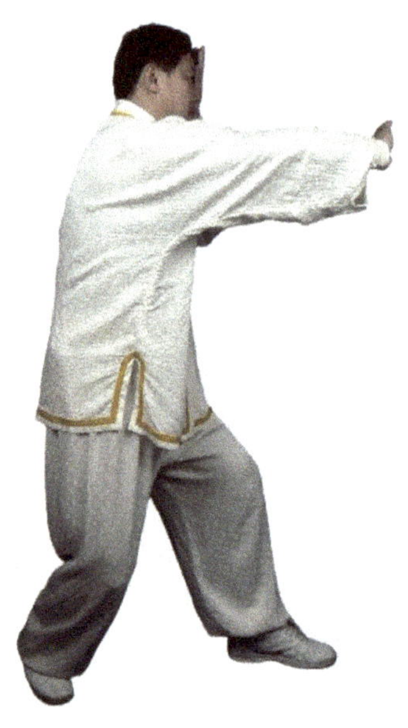

图 9-6 琵琶左势

紧接上动，体微向右转，右臂外旋，右掌回拨，指尖向上，掌心劳宫穴向面部右侧四白穴；左臂内旋，左掌指用力向外弹拨，指尖向右，掌心向前。与之同时，丹田向外凸、缓缓呼气。舌守下腭，牙齿微扣。目随手动意在劳宫穴向四白穴发放热气（图 9-6）。

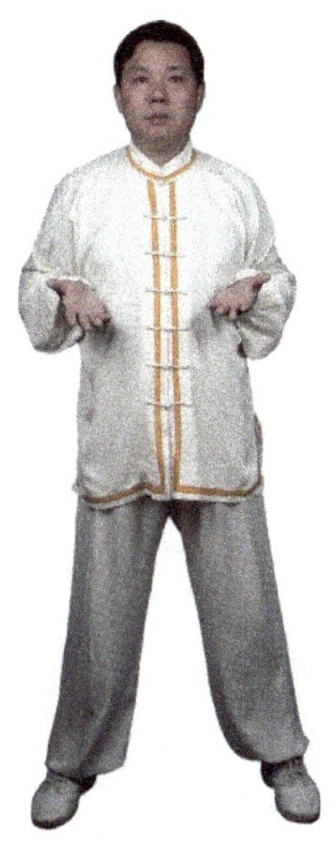

图 9-7 右转合气

4）右转合气

上动略停，身体右转 90 度。调整 2 次呼吸后，两腿伸直，自然站立。同时，两臂外旋，两手随之向内上抬，掌根部停靠于两乳下。指尖向前，掌心向上。与之同时，丹田向内凹、吸气时舌顶上腭，牙齿轻扣，目视前方（图 9-7）。

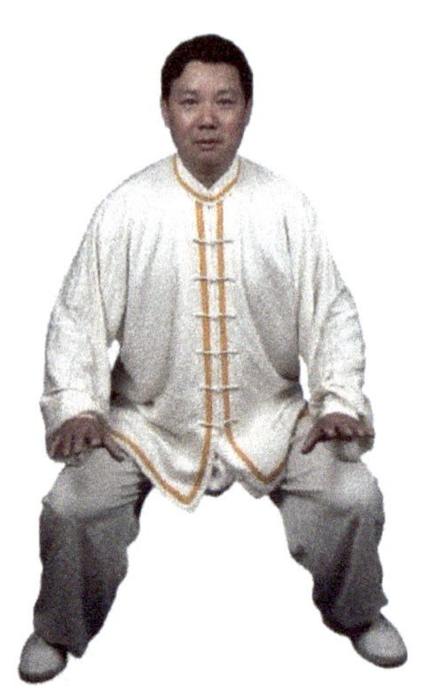

图 9-8 右转合气

上动不停，身体重心下降，两腿屈膝下蹲成马步。同时，两臂内旋，两肘合抱，手向体前弧形下按，停于腹前。掌心向下，指尖向前方。同时，丹田向外凸、呼气。舌守下腭，牙齿微扣。目微下视，意在丹田，气行督任二脉（图 9-8）。

5）琵琶右势

动作方法完全同琵琶左势，惟左右方向相反（参阅图 9-4、9-5、9-6）。

6）转身还原

动作方法完全同推山功无极初开（参阅图 2-1）。上动不停，动作方法完全同无极功混元一气（参阅图 1-8）。

武当气功

要领与功能：

练习琵琶功主要是养肾、强肾。肾主骨，骨生髓，而“脑为髓海”。所以，肾精充足，自然精力充沛，神思敏捷，记忆力强，筋骨强健。

本功动法作，既有舒服松柔，又要大方开展。在相对的放松情况下，全身肌肉、肢节、筋骨、血脉均要伸缩。先后、刚柔必须和谐，周身上下，形成一个整体，连贯协调，动中有静，静中有动。

练习琵琶功，还要注意避免“3 紧”即形体紧、意念紧、呼吸紧。身体在自然中放松，既不可以僵硬呆笨，也不可以软弱无力，做到松而不懈，整个形体有一种内在的气势。

意念要轻盈，若存若息，似守非守，勿望勿助之意，不可强求。呼吸任其自然，舒缓绵绵，不可以憋气，更不能强求、必得。这 3 点要贯穿到练功的全过程中。精气要周流全身经络之间，与动作暗中相合。呼则弹拨，吸则回转。每次行气运功后，还要“还虚入无”收功于下丹田气海穴为要。

如此日积月累，刻苦习练，内部精气运行越来越顺，内气运转的程度越来越高，气体对人体的作用最大。气聚则生，气散则亡。人要长寿，必须爱气息、尊神韵、重精（先天之精和后天之精）。精、气、神充足，则可以达到容颜光彩夺目，耳聪目明，精神饱满，神采奕奕。

武当气功

练习方法：

每次练习以 6 次或 12 次为一组，可以反复习炼。动作的幅度、大小、高低不限，以个人年龄、力量大小、体质强弱而定。

点穴

督脉 GV[who]
任脉 CV[who]
劳宫穴 PC-8[who]
百会穴 GV-20[who]
四白穴 ST-2[who]
气海 CV-6[who]

第十节 抖翎功

运气聚敛汇丹田，
抖翎两翅意外漫。
要认其中玄秘处，
提肛踵息是真传。

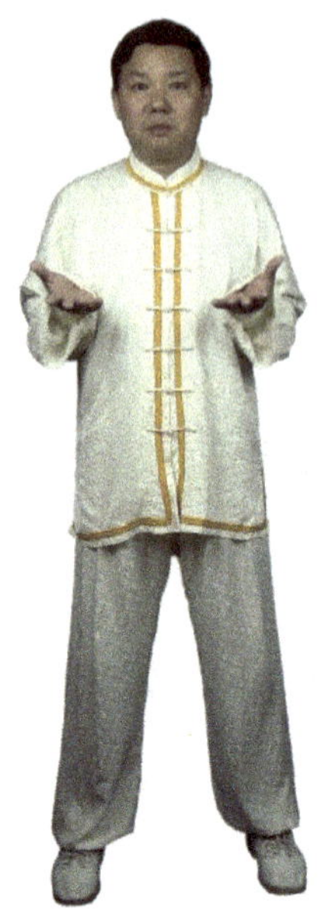

图 10-1 上下调气

1）预备势

动作方法完全同无极功预备势（参阅图 1-1、1-2、1-3、1-4）。

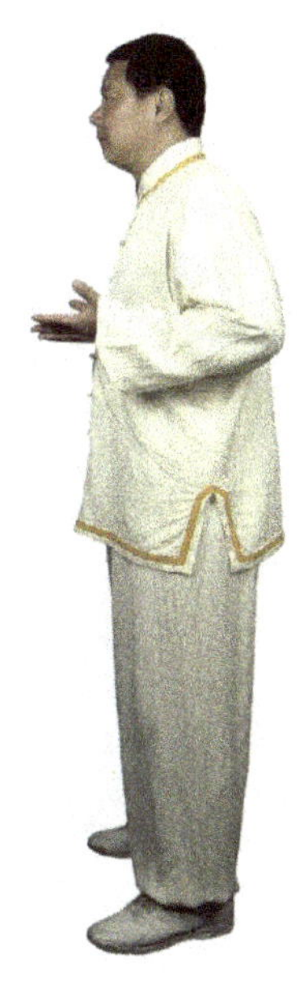

图 10-2 上下调气

2）上下调气

上动略停，调整 2 次呼吸后，两腿伸直，自然站立。同时，两臂外旋，两手随之向内上抬，掌根部停靠于两乳下。双手指尖向前，掌心向上方。同时，丹田向内凹、吸气。舌顶上腭，牙齿轻扣，目视前方（图 10-1、10-2）。

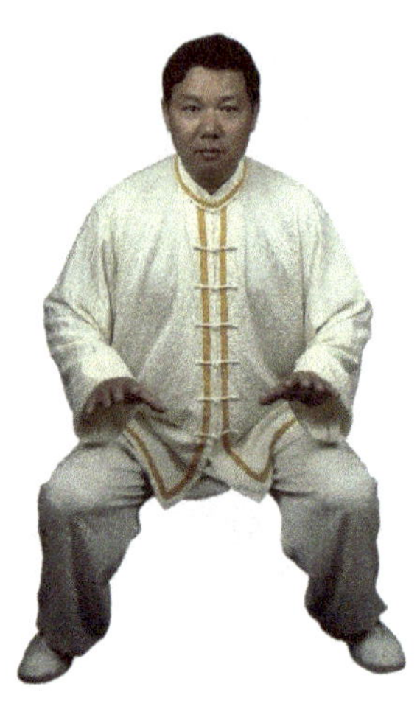

图 10-3 上下调气

上动不停，身体重心下降，两腿屈膝下蹲成马步。同时，两臂内旋，两肘合抱，手向体前弧形下按，停于腹前。掌心向下，指尖向前方。同时，丹田向外凸、呼气。舌守下腭，牙齿微扣。目微下视，意在丹田，气行督任二脉（图 10-3）。

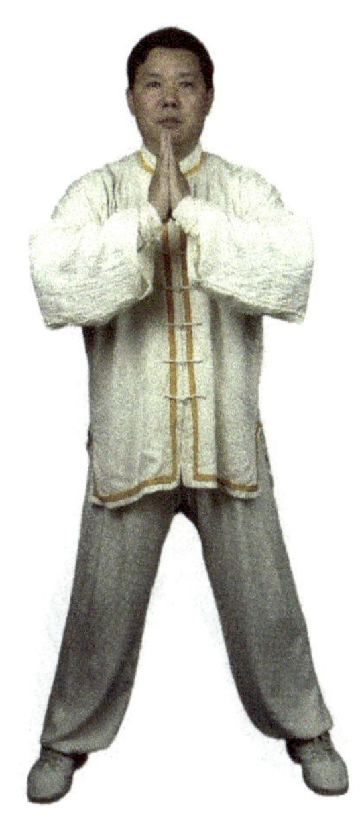

图 10-4 抖翎左势

3）抖翎左势

上动略停，两腿伸直，身体自然站立。同时，两臂外旋上翻，两手向上、向体前抄起，双手合十停于颌前。指尖向上，小指侧向前。同时，丹田向内凹、吸气。舌顶上腭，牙齿轻扣。目微下视，意在头顶百会穴（图 10-4）。

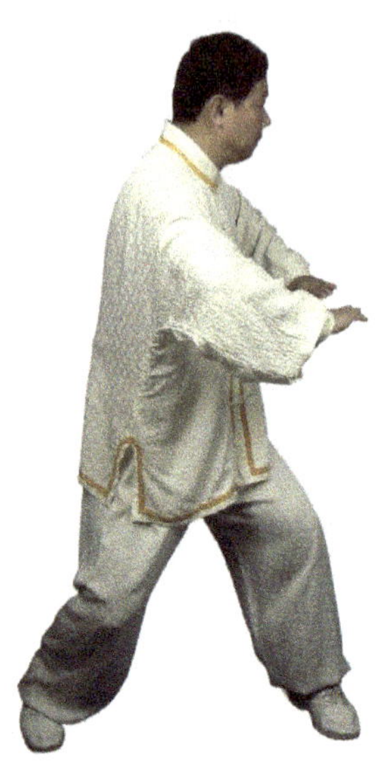

图 10-5 抖翎左势

上动不停，体向左转 90 度，重心为前六后四，成左六四步。同时，两臂内旋，手由胸前分开，向体侧反撑，横抖，略低于髋部。指尖斜向下指，掌心向下，小指一侧向体前。与之同时，丹田向外凸、呼气。舌守下腭，牙齿微扣。目视左下方，意在左小指少冲穴（图 10-5）。

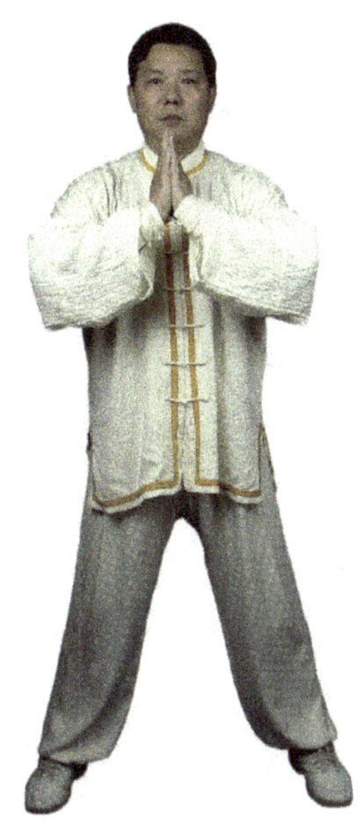

图 10-6 马步右劈

4）马步右劈

上动不停，体向左转 90 度，面南直立。两臂内旋，两手由体侧向上、向体前弧形抄起，双手合十停于颌前。指尖向上指，小指一侧向体前。与之同时，丹田向内凹、吸气。舌顶上腭，牙齿轻扣。目随身移，意在掌心劳宫穴相互吸引（图 10-6）。

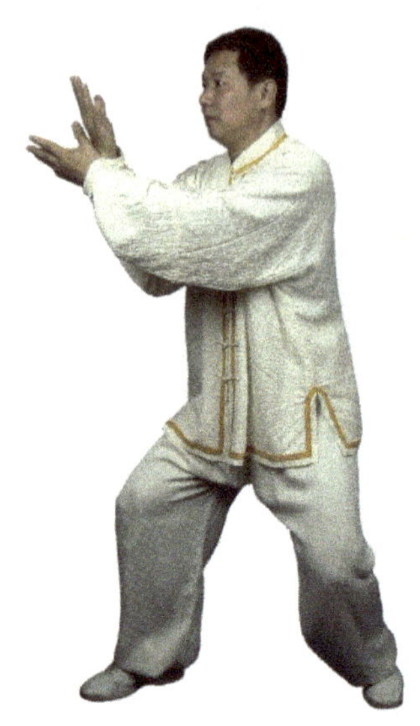

图 10-7 马步右劈

上动略停，体微右转，两腿屈蹲成马步。体微向前倾，两臂外旋，两手由体侧向上、向前弧形抄起，左手指尖向前上，掌心向上；右手停于左腕脉门上方。指尖向左前，掌心向上方。同时，丹田向内凹、吸气。舌顶上腭，牙齿轻扣。目视前下方，意在脚心涌泉穴向上提（图 10-7）。

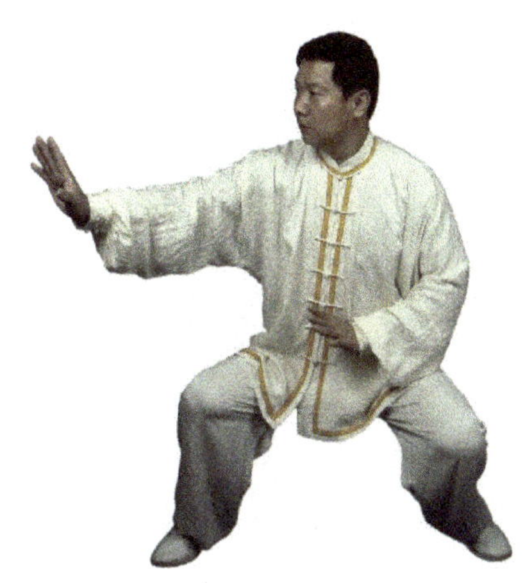

图 10-8 马步右劈

上动不停，体继续向右转 135 度，身体重心下降。同时，右手外缘用力向右前下方劈，与中丹田膻中穴同高，指尖向前上，掌心向前下；左手内旋下压，停于腹前，拇指根节靠于肚脐上，掌心向下，食指上挑，与右手食指相照。劈掌时，丹田向外凸、呼气。舌守下腭，牙齿微扣。目视右手指尖，意在食指少商穴，气行手太阴肺经（图 10-8）。

5）抖翎右势

动作方法完全同抖翎左势，惟左右方向相反（参阅图 10-4、10-5）。

6） 马步左劈

动作方法完全同马步右劈，惟动作方向相反（参阅图10-6、10-7、10-8）。

7） 转体归原

动作方法完全同推山功无极初开（参阅图 2-1）。上动不停，动作方法完全同无极功混元一气（参阅图 1-8）。

要领与功能：

抖翎功练习的的全部过程之中，要刚柔相济，以身领手，以意领气，以气充身，并结合经络循环，使气血均匀分布周身各器官。转动抖翎时，一般采用逆势呼吸，吸则、丹田向内凹；呼则、丹田向外凸。可以使横膈肌下降，呼吸深长，肺活量加大，促使新陈代谢旺盛。重心下移、转身、双肘外顶、双掌撑开的动作要整齐一致。并做到肩松髋合，肘坠膝扣，手撑踵摆。有开有合，先蓄后发。拳经曰："抖翎莫有形，有形必不能。发掌莫带势，带势必不精。"

阴升阳降，清浊转换。一般初习武当气功者，往往口中有痰，下出虚气，此乃是浊气下降，清气上升时的必经过程，属于正常现象。痰要吐出，口内的津液要配合吸气咽入，下降至丹田。古称此为天河水，入丹田者才能水火相济，明润心肾。

武当气功

练习中意念务必专注，有杂念出现时，心中要暗念 8 法：

- 心定神宁、
- 神宁心安、
- 心安清静、
- 清静无物、
- 无物气行、
- 气行绝相、
- 绝相觉明、
- 觉明则神气相通，万象归根 。

练习方法：

每次练习以 6 次或 12 次为一组，可以反复练习。动作的幅度大小、高低不限，以个人的年龄、力量大小、体质强弱而定。

点穴

督脉 GV[who]
任脉 CV[who]
百会穴 GV-20[who]
少冲穴 HT-9[who]
劳宫穴 PC-8[who]
脉门 HT-9[who]
涌泉穴 KC-1[who]

第十一节　白猿献果功

白猿承浆奉仙果，
老君赐丹在炉前。
种瓜种豆非枉然，
外伸内收自成仙。

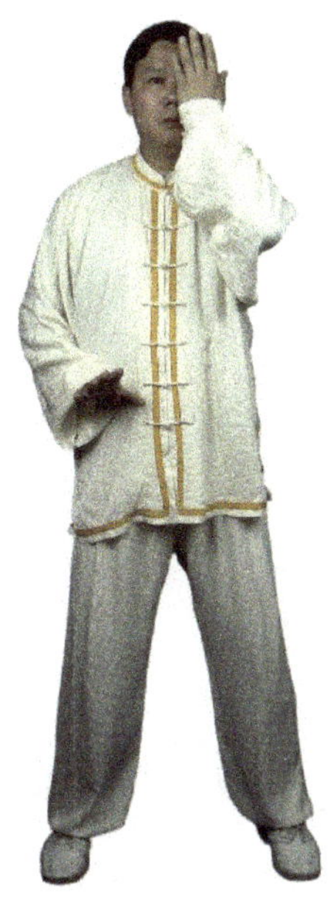

图 11-1 猿猴洗脸

1）预备势

动作方法完全同无极功预备势（参阅图 1-1、1-2、1-3、1-4）。

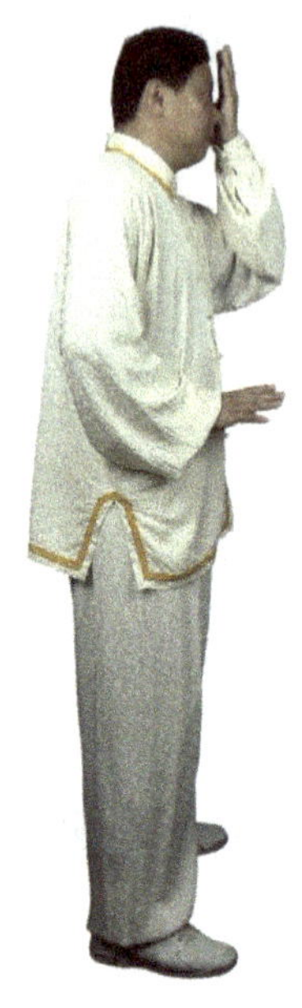

图 11-2 猿猴洗脸

2）猿猴洗脸

上动略停，左臂外旋，左手由体侧抄起，停于左眼角外侧，指尖向上，掌心向内。左手劳宫穴用意下摩向左面部发功；右手随之向上抬，停于腰间带脉处，指尖向前，掌心向下。与之同时，丹田向内凹、吸气。舌顶上腭，牙齿轻扣。目微闭合，意在左掌，气行足少阳胆经（图 11-1、11-2）。

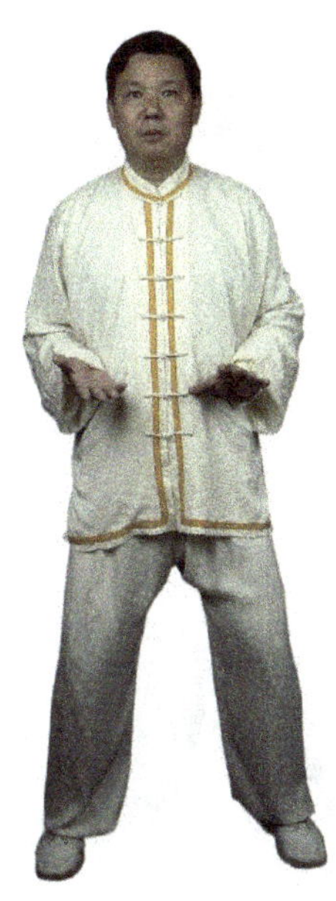

图 11-3 猿猴洗脸

上动不停，身体重心下降，两腿屈膝下蹲成马步。同时，左臂内旋，左掌心劳宫穴用意向下顺身体左侧发功，停于腰间带脉部，指尖向前，掌心向下成阴掌。同时，右臂外旋，右掌翻转成阳掌停于腰间，指间向前，掌心向上方。同时，丹田向外凸、呼气。舌守下腭，牙齿微扣。目视前方，意在丹田，气循行带脉（图 11-3）。

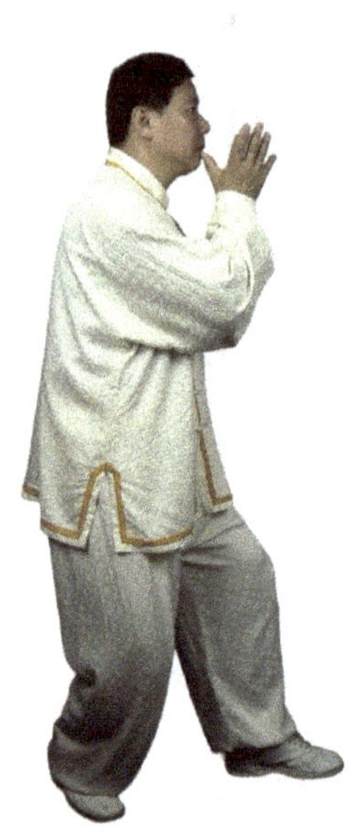

图 11-4 献果左势

3）献果左势

上动略停，身体重心移至右腿，体向左转 90 度。左脚尖翘起，右脚跟着地成左高虚步。两掌由腰间向面部弧形上托，如捧物状。掌根部靠拢，指间斜向上方，两手拇指相倚对着下颌承浆穴。与之同时，丹田向内凹、吸气。舌顶上腭，牙齿轻扣。目随身移，意在涌泉穴，气行太阴肺经（图 11-4）。

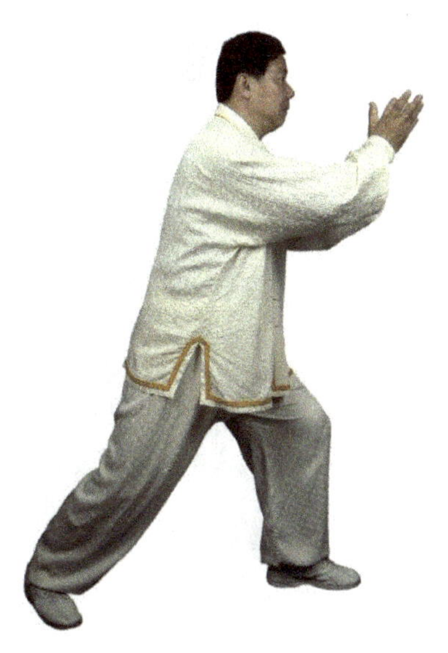

图 11-5 献果左势

上动不停，左脚向前垫半步，全脚着地，左腿屈蹲；右腿挺膝伸直成左弓步。同时，双手由承浆穴处向上、向左前方弧形推出，两臂伸直，略高于眼。5 指自然伸开，虎口撑圆，拇指尖向上，其余 4 指向前。与之同时，丹田向外凸、呼气。舌守下腭，牙齿微扣。目随手上视，意在掌心劳宫穴，气行手厥阴心包经（图 11-5）。

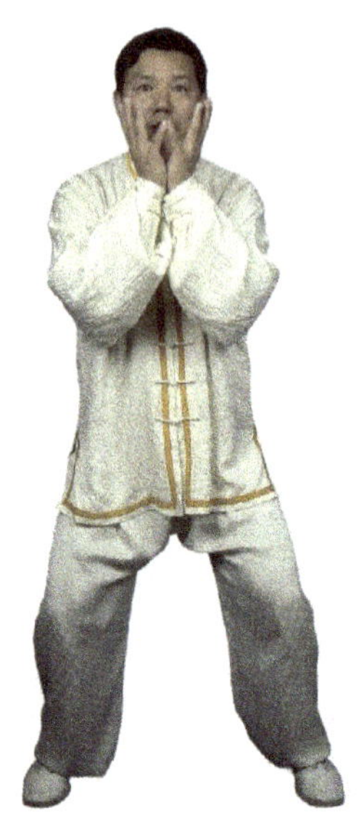

图 11-6 收果内敛

4）收果内敛

上动略停，身体向右转 90 度。左脚微向回收，身体重心升起，自然站立。同时，两掌回挂，双手捧果停于颌下。小指外侧向前，掌根靠拢停于玉堂穴边。与之同时，丹田向内凹、吸气。舌顶上腭，牙齿轻扣。目微下视，意在玄关窍处（图 11-6）。

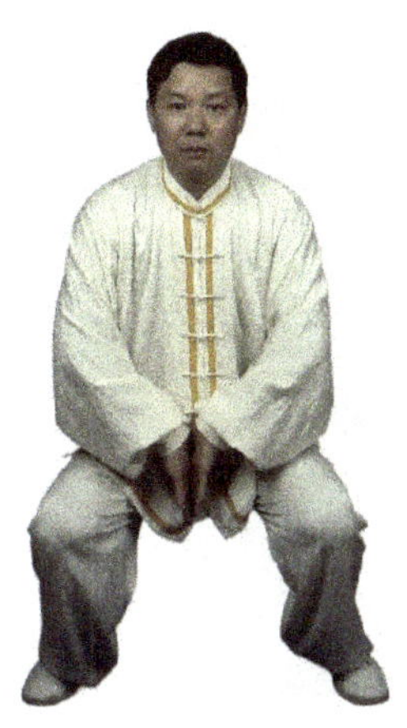

图 11-7 收果内敛

上动不停，身体重心下降，两腿屈膝下蹲成马步。同时，两臂内旋，肩松肘坠，两掌由胸前翻转下插，停于腹下丹田处，指尖向下，手背相贴，小指侧向前。与之同时，丹田向外凸、呼气。舌守下腭，牙齿微扣。目视前方，意在精气下行丹田（图 11-7、11-8）。

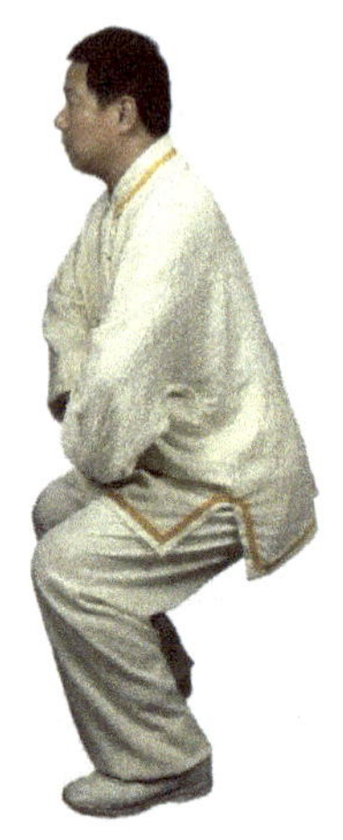

图 11-8 猿猴洗脸

5） 猿猴洗脸

动作方法完全同前猿猴洗脸，惟左右方向相反（参阅图 11-1、11-2、11-3）。

6） 献果右势

动作方法完全同献果左势，惟左右方向相反（参阅图 11-4、11-5）。

7）转身小收

动作方法完全同推山功无极初开（参阅图 2-1）。上动不停，动作方法完全同无极功混元一气（参阅图 1-8）。

武当气功

要领与功能

白猿献果功以屈曲伸缩翻转压气、津液还丹、气息循行带脉为主。带脉横行于腰、腹之间，它将全身直行的各经络约束起来，为一条带子。有总束诸经络，使之不能妄行的作用。意念要着重 3 守：1 守和，就是指“万物负阴而抱阳，冲气为和”，故要守和。 2 守神，就是指“人之耳目，何能久劳而不息；人之精神，何能驰骋而不乏”，故需内守不失。 3 守气，就是指“血气专忽而不越外，则胸腹气充盈意专注”，故当守气。做到 3 守则人平和，神安宁、气运行。

两手体前捧果，5 指要分开外撑，向前推 进时，一定要向上弧形运动。这样就会逐步起到“扶正驱邪”的作用。扶正驱邪的“正”就是正气、浩然气，是指人体抵抗疾病，维护健康的能力；“邪”就是邪气，是各种致病的因素。人生病，就是正气不足，邪气入侵或邪气太盛所致。先师曰：“正气内守”，“邪安从来”。而“扶正”能增强上体机能的抵抗力。

练习方法：

每次练习以 6 次或 12 次为一组，可以反腹练习。动作的幅度大小、高低不限，以个人的年龄、力量大小、体质强弱而定。

武当气功

点穴

劳宫穴 PC-8[who]

带脉 GB-26[who]

足少阳胆经 GB[who]

承浆穴 CV-24[who]

涌泉穴 KC-1[who]

手太阴肺经 LU[who]

厥阴心包经 PC[who]

玉堂穴 CV-18[who]

玄关窍

第十二节 丹凤朝阳功

丹凤朝阳气通天，
肩松肘坠辩阴阳。
呼吸行功和术数，
百年长寿乐安康。

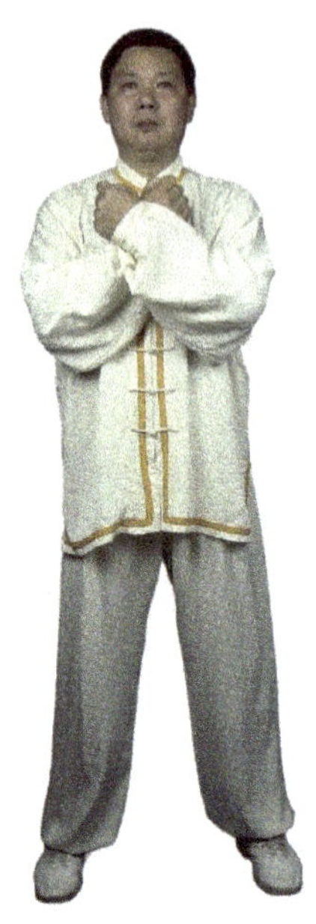

图 12-1 起钻落翻

1）预备势

动作方法完全同无极功预备势（参阅图 1-1、1-2、1-3、1-4）。

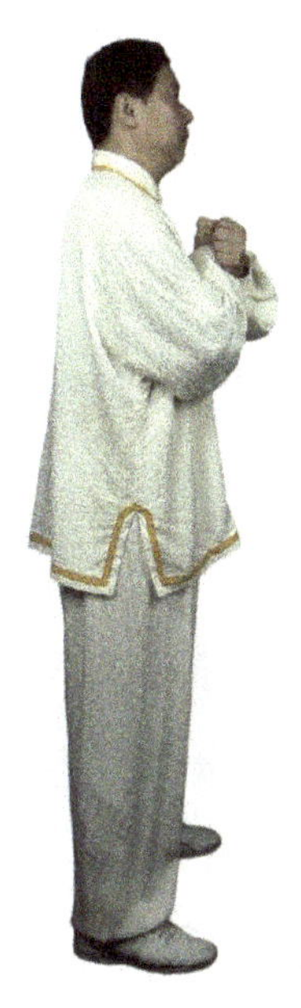

图 12-2 起钻落翻

2） 起钻落翻

上动略停，两臂外旋，两掌变拳由体侧向上、向前弧形上钻。左拳在外；右拳在内，十字交叉，停于胸前。拳背向前，拳心向内，掌根大陵穴对胸侧周荣穴。同时，丹田向内凹、吸气。舌顶上腭，牙齿轻扣。目微合闭，意在百会穴，气行足太阴脾经（图 12-1、12-2）。

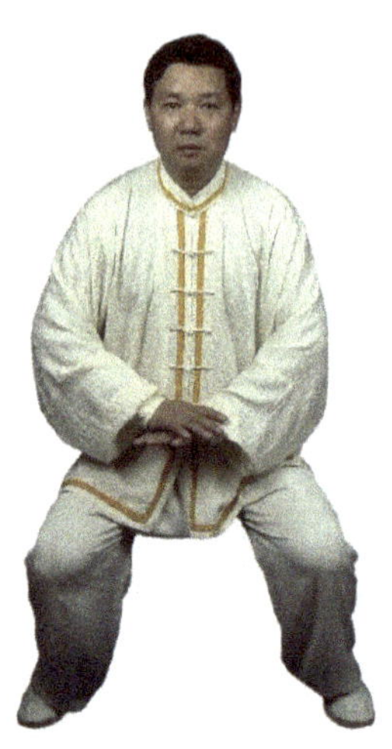

图 12-3 起钻落翻

上动不停，上体重心下降，两腿屈膝下蹲成马步。同时，两臂内旋，两拳变掌向腹前按压（右上、左下）。指尖斜向前方，掌心向前下。与之同时，丹田向外凸、呼气。目视前下方，意在食指上挑（图 12-3）。

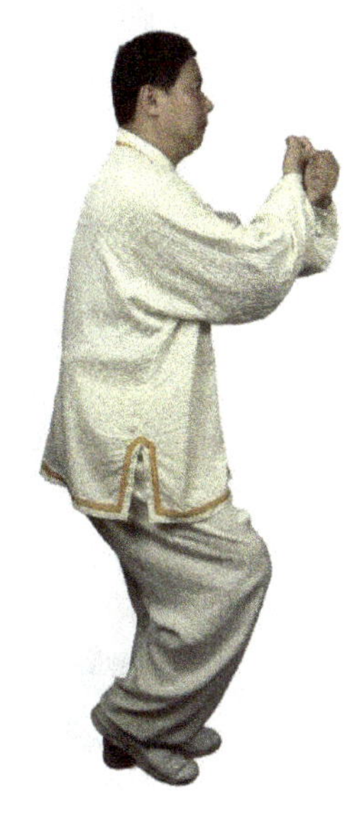

图 12-4 丹凤左势

3）丹凤左势

上动略停，上体重心移至左腿，身体左转 90 度，面向东方。右脚前移至左脚脚弓处，脚尖点地成右丁步。同时，两臂外旋，双手 10 指屈曲成拳，由腹前向前上方弧形上钻，右拳在内；左拳在外，十字交叉停于胸前。右小臂内关穴压在左下臂外关穴上，拳背向前，拳心向后。同时，丹田向内凹、吸气。舌顶上腭，牙齿轻扣。目随身转，意在内关外关穴（图 12-4）。

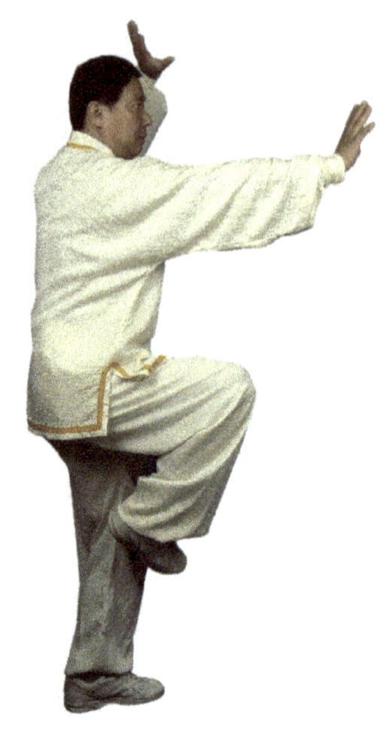

图 12-5 丹凤左势

上动不停，左腿直立支撑，右腿屈提，脚尖向下成右独立势。提腿同时，两臂内旋，双手 10 指伸开成掌。左掌由胸前向上弧形划弧屈肘上架，横停于头顶上方，指尖向右，掌心向上；右掌用力向前缓缓推出，指尖向上，掌心向前。架推同时，丹田向外凸、呼气。舌守下腭，牙齿微扣。目视前手掌，意在双掌撕拉（图 12-5）。

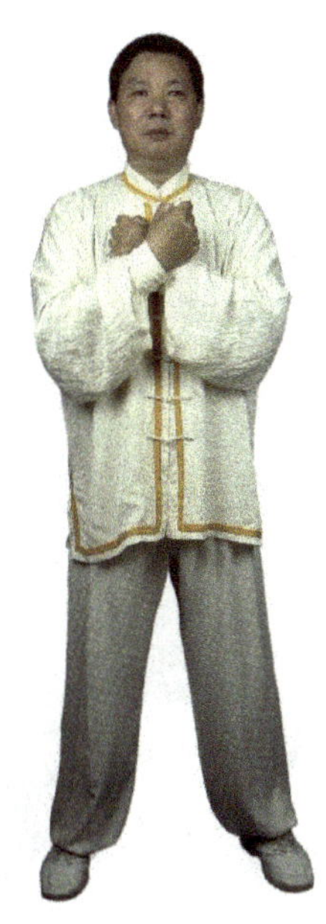

图 12-6 转身合气

4）转身合气

上动略停，右脚向后下方落地，身体右转 90 度，面向南方。两臂外旋，两掌变拳由体侧向上向前弧形上钻。右拳在外；左拳在内，十字交叉停于胸前。拳背向前，拳心向内，掌根大陵穴对着胸侧周荣穴。与之同时，丹田向内凹、吸气。舌顶上腭，牙齿轻扣。目微合闭，意在百会穴，气行足太阴脾经（图 12-6）。

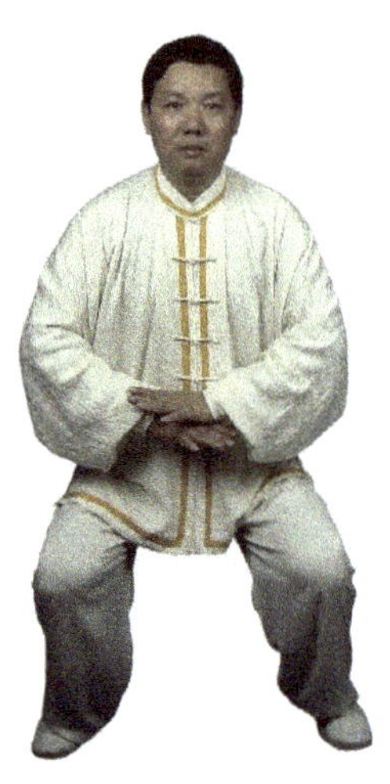

图 12-7 转身合气

上动不停，上体重心下降，两腿屈膝下蹲成马步。同时，两臂内旋，两拳变掌向腹前按压（左上、右下）。指尖斜向前，掌心向下。与之同时，丹田向外凸、呼气。目视前下方，意在食指上挑（图 12-7）。

5）朝阳右势

动作方法完全同丹凤左势，惟左右方向相反（参阅图 12-4、12-5）。

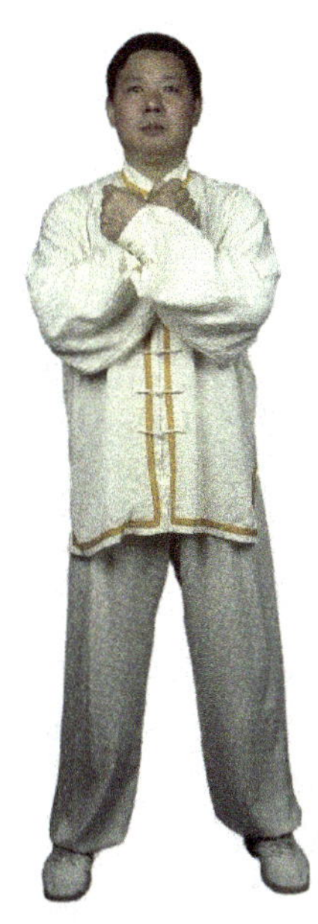

图 12-8 回身收势

6）回身收势

上动略停，左脚向后下落地，身体左转 90 度，面向南方，自然站立。同时两臂外旋，两掌变拳收回，左拳在外右拳在内，十字交叉停于胸前，拳背向前，拳心向内。与之同时，丹田向内凹、吸气。舌顶上腭，牙齿轻扣。目随身转，意在胸侧周荣穴（图 12-8）。

动作方法完全同无极功混元一气（参阅图 1-8）。

武当气功

要领与功能：

丹凤朝阳功主要是“炼精化气”，内气运行大小周天。转体时，以腰带动周身一齐转动，双手胸前斜十字交叉，掌心劳宫穴与胸侧周荣穴相对，互相吸引。提腿独立与上架前的推掌要协调，合拍。身体必须保持平稳，周身放松稍含胸。落步、对拳与重心下降整齐一致，要持之以恒不断习练。练到一定程度时，就会感到，呼气时气从丹田经会阴穴直达涌泉穴；吸气时，气从涌泉经会阴到命门，这样长强穴自然就会通顺。接下去就要气通夹脊穴、玉枕穴。夹脊在大椎下 9 厘米处，玉枕在脑后风府穴下。

初练时，会感到脊椎发木，后感到发胀、发麻、发热，最后，气由命门直贯夹脊处。待夹脊处气感达到 6 厘米宽时，夹脊穴就可以通顺了。而后，用此法通顺玉枕穴，待玉枕穴处气感达到 6 厘米宽时，玉枕穴也通了。

在这个基础上，则可以使气向上行达于百会穴，这时感到一股热带向上流，按摩小脑，头顶感到清凉湿润，全身舒服无比。然后气向下降，经两眼和鼻部向下行至人中穴。此时将顶上腭的舌下落于下腭，微微扣牙齿，气就下行至承浆穴，使督任二脉接通，气从任脉下归于丹田。如果在练功时发生舌枯口干、心烦、意燥等上火现象，意念就要移至涌泉穴、命门穴，会阴穴，使之阴阳相合，水火相济。完成此步功夫，就可以防病祛病。

武当气功

练习方法：

每次练习以 6 次或 12 次为一组，可以反复练习。动作的幅度大小、高低不限，以个人的年龄、力量大小、体质强弱而定。

点穴

内关 PC-6[who]
大陵穴 PC-7[who]
周荣穴 SP-20[who]
百会穴 GV-20[who]
太阴脾经 SP[who]
外关 TB-5
大陵穴 PC-7[who]
周荣穴 SP-20[who]
太阴脾经 SP[who]
劳宫穴 PC-8[who]
会阴 CV-1[who]
涌泉穴 KC-1[who]
命门穴 GV-4[who]
夹脊穴
玉枕 BK-9[who]
风府穴 GV-16[who]
人中穴 GV-26[who]
承浆穴 CV-24[who]
任脉 CV[who]
长强穴 GV-1[who]

第十三节　拨草寻蛇功

腋底藏花不为奇，
左摆右扣乃为宜。
拨草寻蛇右兮左，
意气相随固根基。

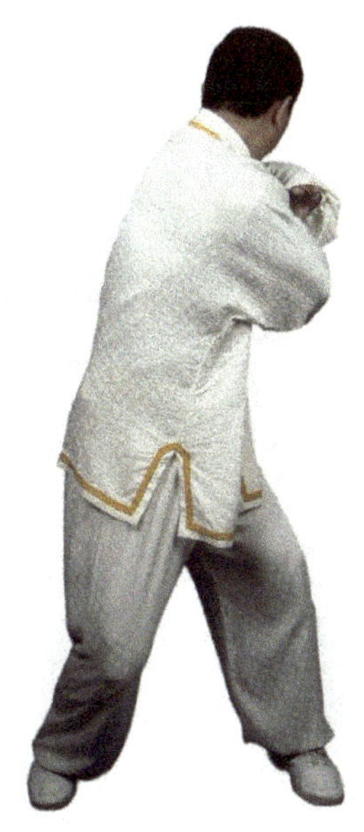

图 13-1 拨草寻蛇左势

1）预备势

动作方法完全同无极功预备势（参阅图 1-1、1-2、1-3、1-4）。

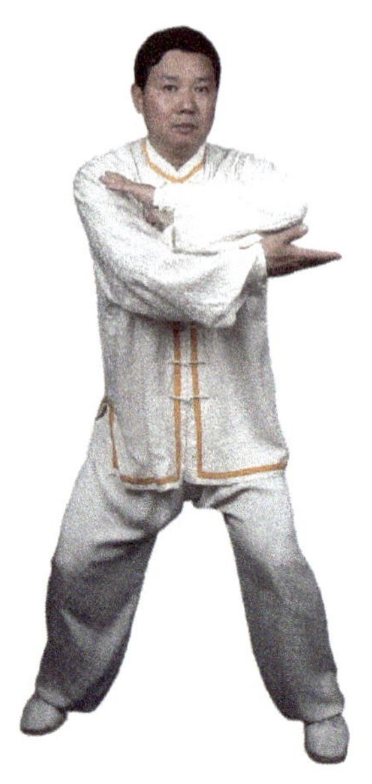

图 13-2 拨草寻蛇左势

2）拨草寻蛇左势

上动略停，右脚尖内扣，身体重心落于两腿之间，成弓马步。右臂外旋，右手由体侧向左上方穿，停于左腋下，指尖向左，掌心向上方，手心劳宫穴对着腋下极泉穴；左手向右上方划弧，停于右肘关节上侧，指尖向右，掌心向下。与之同时，丹田向内凹、吸气。舌顶上腭，牙齿轻扣。目视左前方，意在气贯百会穴（图 13-1、13-2）。

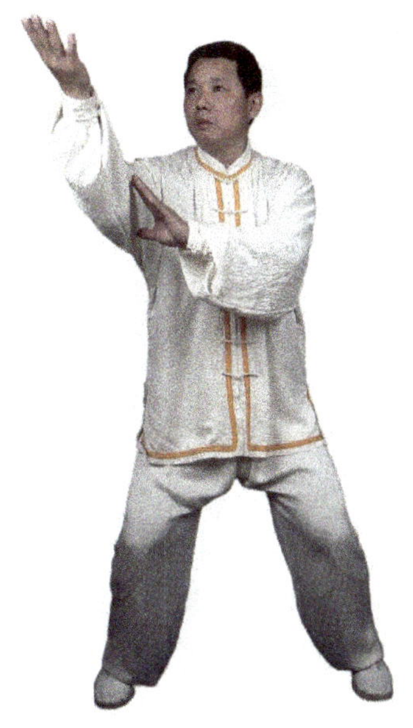

图 13-3 拨草寻蛇左势

上动不停，身体重心上升，体向右转，两臂向右前上方摆出。右手在上略高于头；左手在下与鼻同高，停于右肘关节上侧。双手指尖向前上方，手背向下。同时，丹田向外凸、呼气。舌守下腭，牙齿微扣。目视右手，意在下臂孔最穴，气血循行手太阴肺经（图 13-3）。

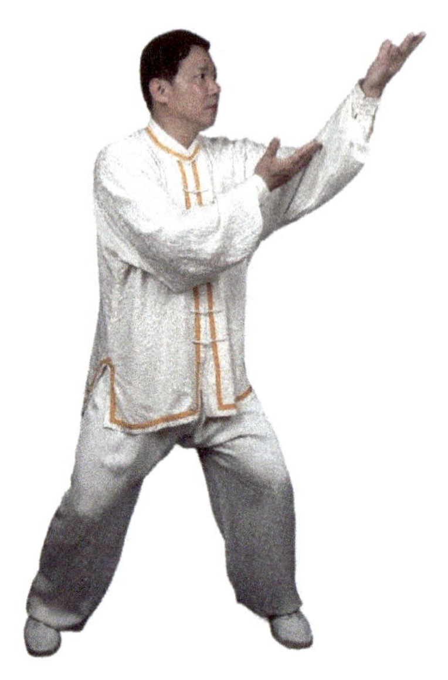

图 13-4 拨草寻蛇左势

上动略停，体向左转，两臂内旋，小指一侧的手臂用力翻转，双手腕部交叉成十字手，右下、左上停于头左侧，掌心向内上方，指尖斜向上方。与之同时，丹田向内凹、吸气。舌顶上腭，牙齿轻扣。目随掌转，意在腕部神门穴（图 13-4）。

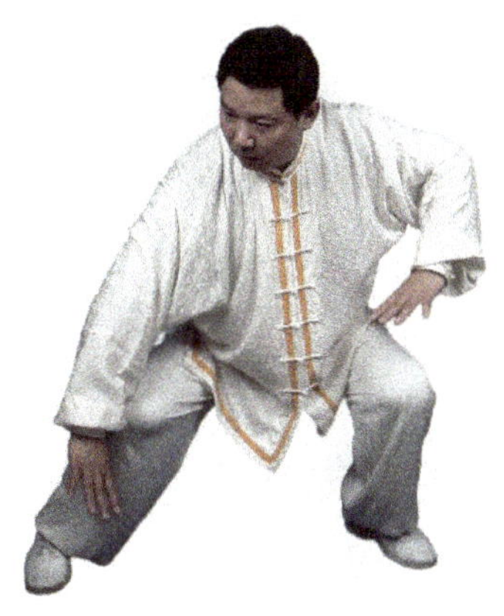

图 13-5 拨草寻蛇左势

上动不停，休向左转。身休重心下降，左腿屈膝下蹲，右腿向右跨半步成右横四六步。同时，两肘关节外撑，双手向下用力按压，而后，再向两侧分拨，停于膝下。掌心向下，小指一侧向前。与之同时，丹田向外凸、呼气。舌守下腭，牙齿微扣。目视前下方，意在双手拨草寻蛇，气血循行阳明大肠经（图 13-5）。

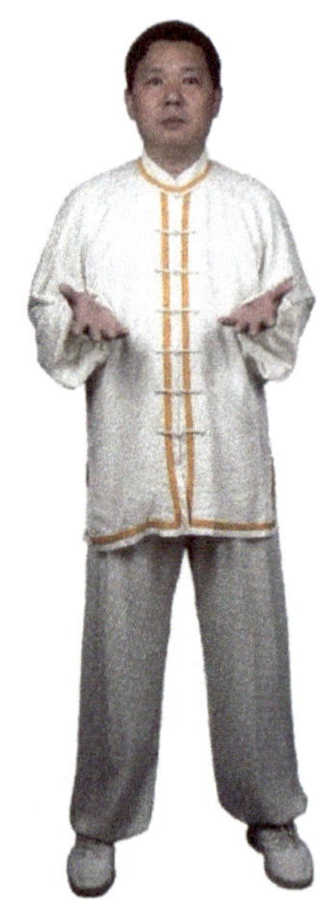

图 13-6 立身小收

3）立身小收

上动略停，体向右转，仍面向南方。调整 2 次呼吸后，两腿伸直，自然站立。同时，两臂外旋，两手随之向内上抬，掌根部停靠于两乳下。双手指尖向前，掌心向上。与之同时，丹田向内凹、吸气。舌顶上腭，牙齿轻扣，目视前方（图 13-6）。

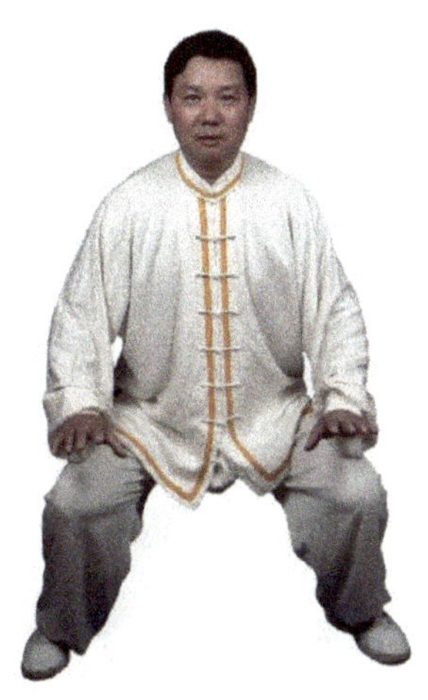

图 13-7 立身小收

上动不停，身体重心下降，两腿屈膝下蹲成马步，同时，两臂内旋，两肘合抱，手向体前弧形下按，停于腹前。掌心向下，指尖向前方。同时，丹田向外凸、呼气。舌守下腭，牙齿微扣。目微下视，意在丹田，气行督任二脉（图 13-7, 13-8）。

4）拨草寻蛇右势

动作方法完全同拨草寻蛇左势，惟左右方向相反（参阅图 13-1、13-2、13-3、13-4、13-5）。

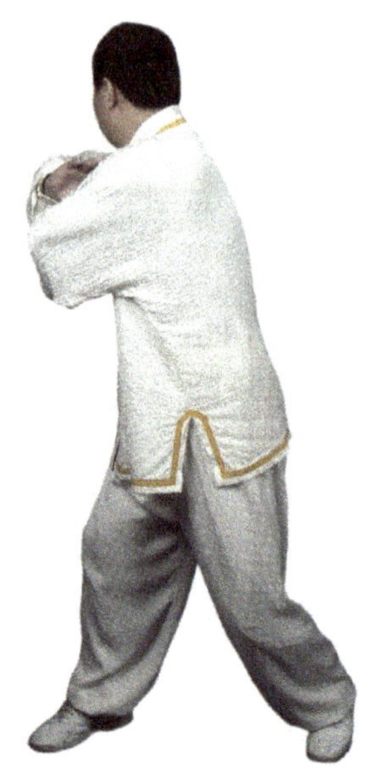

图 13-8 拨草寻蛇右势

5）起身还原

动作方法完全同推山功无极初开（参阅图 2-1）。上动不停，动作方法完全同无极功混元一气（参阅图 1-8）。

武当气功

要领与功能

拨草寻蛇功，主要练习聚神意坚，下盘根基稳固。做到髋要松、要缩，膝要扣、要活，足要平稳，运行练功中手脚要一致、和顺。手占 3 分力，足用 7 分劲，五营四梢要合全，气随心意任我行，拨草寻蛇灵气升。

聚神意坚，就是在练功中不能有杂念。一旦杂念出现了，如何排除呢？就是要聚神于一念，以一念代万念，并不是不要任何意念。当然，从一开始的心猿意马，练到心定神宁，神宁心安，心头波平水静的境界，是需要一个复杂的泛化过程的。如果杂念一出现，就手忙脚乱，就发急，或者干脆不练了，是一辈子也练不好的。众所周知，克服杂念的过程，就是功夫长进有收益的过程。一定要把意念守在功法中所要求的经络、部位、或某个穴位。天长日久就做到了聚神意坚，以一念代万念代杂念。

精于拳术气功者都懂得，下盘不可松懈。下盘松懈浑身落空，似浮萍无根。练功至根深蒂固，运变灵活，才能处处落实。功法中要求的一切松静园活，都是从根里生出来的。如果能牢牢地掌握这一原则，自然而然就能达到化境。

练习方法

每次练习以 6 次或 12 次为一组，可以反 复练习。动作的幅度大小、高低不限，以个人的年龄、力量大小、体质强弱而定。

武当气功

点穴

劳宫穴 PC-8[who]

极泉穴 HT-1[who]

百会穴 GV-20[who]

孔最 LU-6[who]

手太阴肺经 LU[who]

神门穴 HT-7[who]

手阳明大肠经 LI[who]

督脉 GV[who]

任脉 CV[who]

第十四节 龙虎相交功

西山白虎放颠狂，
东方青龙不可当。
龙虎相交金合木，
性情自伏而成丹。

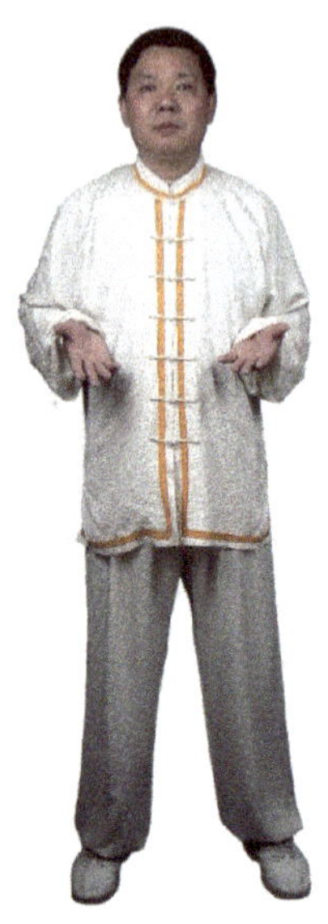

图 14-1 金木相合

1）预备势

动作方法完全同无极功预备势（参阅图 1-1、1-2、1-3、1-4）。

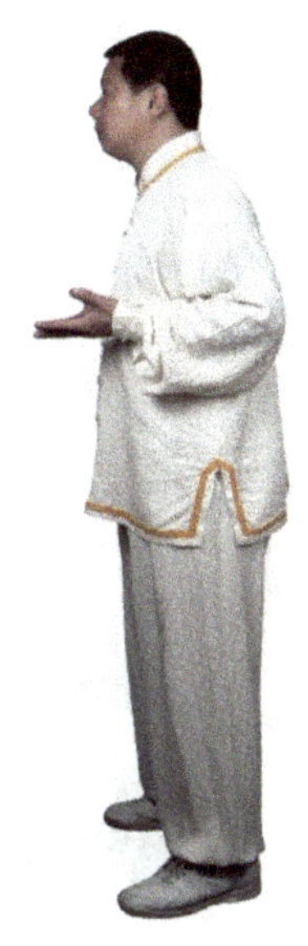

图 14-2 金木相合

2）金木相合

上动略停，调整 2 次呼吸后，两腿伸直自然站立。同时，两臂外旋，两手随之向上抬，掌根部停靠于两乳下。双手指尖向前，掌心向上。同时，丹田向内凹、吸气。舌顶上腭，牙齿轻扣，目视前方（图 14-1、14-2 ）。

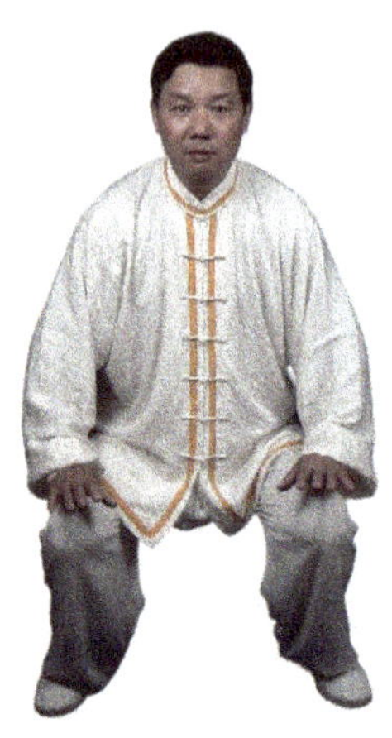

图 14-3 金木相合

上动不停，身体重心下降，两腿屈膝下蹲成马步。同时，两臂内旋，两肘合抱，手向体前弧形下按，停于腹前。掌心向下，指尖向前方。同时，丹田向外凸、呼气。舌守下腭，牙齿微扣。目微下视，意在丹田，气行督任二脉（图 14-3）。

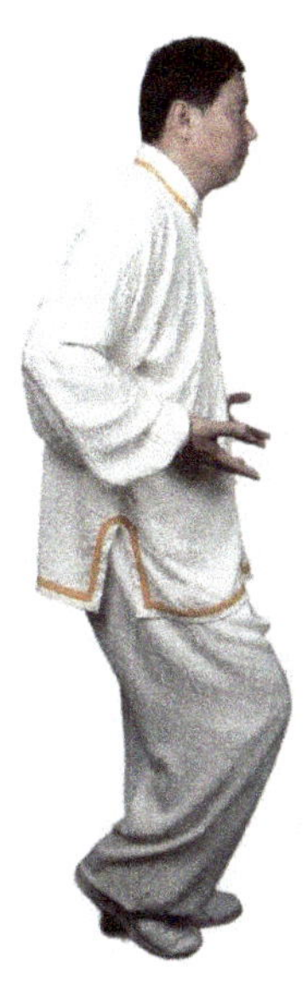

图 14-4 龙虎相交左势

3）龙虎相交左势

上动略停，体向左转 90 度，左腿屈蹲，右脚随之跟进，停于左脚内侧，脚尖点地，身体重心落于左脚成右丁步。同时，两掌由脐下向左前方弧形上托，停于胸前中庭穴处。两手中指相倚，指尖斜指前下，掌心向内上方。与之同时，丹田向内凹、吸气。舌顶上腭，牙齿轻扣。目随身移，意在食指商阳穴，气行手阳明大肠经（图 14-4）。

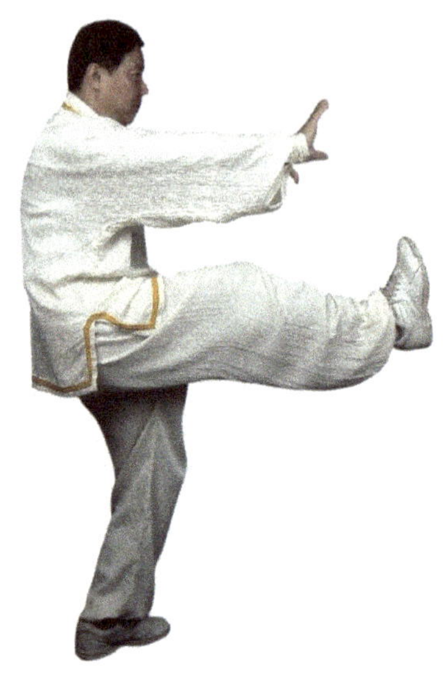

图 14-5 龙虎相交左势

上动不停，左腿挺膝伸直；右腿屈提，脚底用力向前蹬出，与髋同高，脚尖向上，脚心向前。同时，两臂向内旋，以肩催肘，以肘顶腕，肩、肘、腕 3 关节一齐用力使手掌向前推出，与肩同高。指尖相对，掌心向前。同时，丹田向外凸、呼气。舌守下腭，牙齿微扣。目从手指间远视，意在心肾相交（图 14-5）。

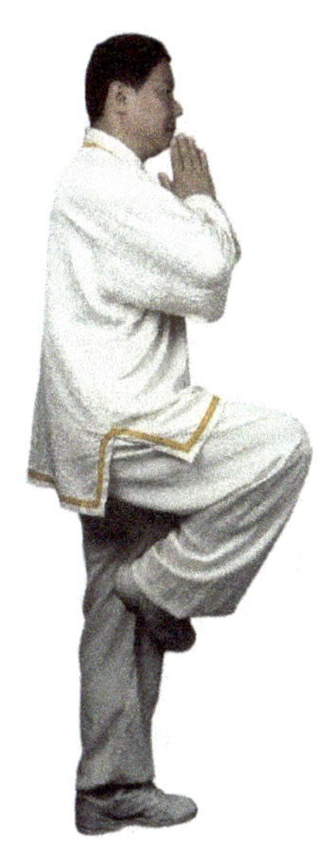

图 14-6 金鸡独立

4）金鸡独立

上动略停，左腿伸直支撑身体；右腿屈膝回收脚尖向下，脚面绷直成右独立势。同时，两臂微向外旋，双掌根合拢，拇指尖靠停于唇下承浆穴处。指尖向上，小指一侧向前。与之同时，丹田向内凹、吸气。舌顶上腭，牙齿轻扣。目视前下方，意在上唇人中穴，气由督脉而上至头顶（图 14-6）。

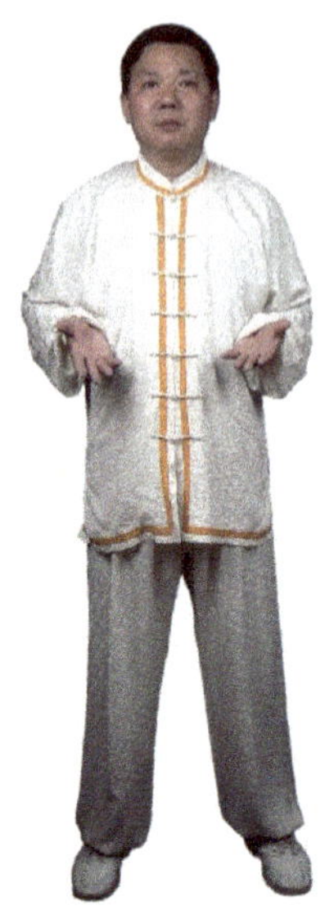

图 14-7 金鸡独立

上动不停，身体右转 90 度。右腿落地，左脚尖内扣，面向南方自然站立。动作方法完全同无极功混元一气（图 14-7）。

5）龙虎相交右势

动作方法完全同龙虎相交左势，惟左右方向相反（参阅图 14-4、14-5）。

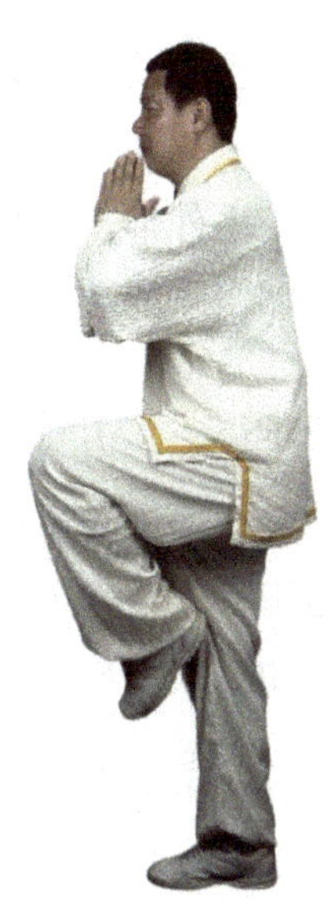

图 14-8 独立收势

6）独立收势

上动略停，右腿伸直支撑身体，左腿屈膝回收，脚尖向下，脚面绷直成左独立势。与之同时，两臂微向外旋，两掌合拢，食指尖顶着鼻下人中穴，指尖向上，小指一侧向前。与之同时，丹田向内凹、吸气。舌顶上腭，牙齿轻扣。目微下视，意在人中穴，气由督脉上升至头顶（图 14-8）。

动作方法完全同无极功混元一气（参阅图 1-8）。

武当气功

要领与功能：

龙虎相交功的练习过程中，要时刻做到心与意相合、意与气相合、气与力（动作）相结合。提腿独立、阴掌下按与呼吸拍节暗合，蹬腿与双手外推，要整齐一致。总而言之，一肢动，百肢齐摇。静如山岳威严挺立，动如迅雷不及掩耳。以心神统领意念，守穴位、部位；以意念统领内气，循行小小周天、小周天、大周天；内气运行与功法动作要求相合，力断意不断，意断气相连。丹田内凹，提肾水上行于脑，向前下撞玄关窍达于心，使心火、肾水相济，而下落于丹田，丹田充盈而体坚如石。

“虎”、比喻元精，元精生于肾气之中。肾属坎卦，属水，有“虎向水边生”之说。

“龙”、比喻元神，元神生于心液之中。心属离卦，属火，有“龙从火里出”之说。

又谓人之本性属木，木位于东方，于卦为震，于人体属肝，故也称之为青龙；情为人的情欲，属金，金位于西方，于卦为兑，于人体属肺，故也称之谓白虎。以五行相克论之，金能克木，因此，情欲往往损伤本性。练习龙虎相交功时，要以真意来克制，去降龙伏虎，使之交合为一。则金木无间，性情自伏而炼成金丹。通过意念的集中，思想上的入静，机体的放松，达到调养心神，心气则可以发挥统辖血液运动的功能。经过本功法练习，精气充足，不但“由元阴”、“元阳”可以互济互根，而且肾水还可以与心火相济，因心肾不交而造成的心悸失眠、遗精等症状，也可以得到改善。而且心脏协调脏腑的功能也可以随之而加强。

武当气功

练习方法：

每次练习以 6 次或 12 次为一组，可以反复练习。动作的幅度大小、高低不限，以个人年龄、力量大小、体质强弱而定。

点穴

督脉 GV[who]

任脉 CV[who]

中庭穴 CV-16[who]

商阳穴 LI-1[who]

手阳明大肠经 LI[who]

承浆穴 CV-24[who]

人中穴 GV-26[who]

玄关窍

第十五节 蛇盘功

蛇盘功叠系一根，
鼻端细息似绵锦。
炼成百宝如意丹，
以精化气气养身。

武当气功

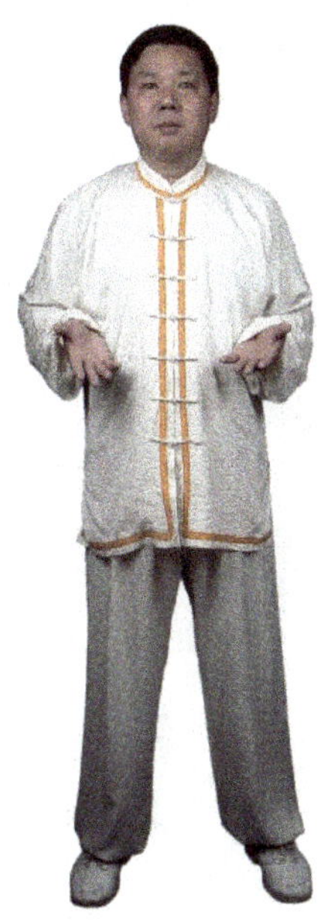

图 15-1 上下调气

1）预备势

动作方法完全同无极功预备势（参阅图 1-1、1-2、1-3、1-4）。

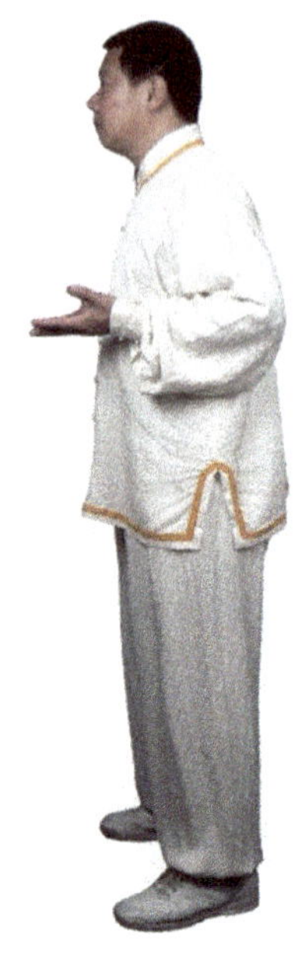

图 15-2 上下调气

2）上下调气

上动略停，调整 2 次呼吸后，两腿伸直，自然站立。同时，两臂外旋，两手随之向内上抬，掌根部停靠于两乳下。双手指尖向前，掌心向上方。同时，丹田向内凹、吸气。舌顶上腭，牙齿轻扣，目视前方（图 15-1、15-2）。

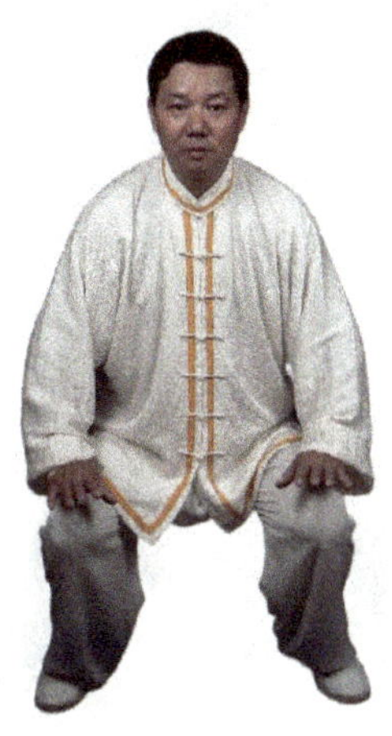

图 15-3 上下调气

上动不停，身体重心下降，两腿屈膝下蹲成马步。同时，两臂内旋，两肘合抱，手向体前弧形下按，停于腹前。掌心向下，指尖向前方。同时，丹田向外凸、呼气。舌守下腭，牙齿微扣。目微下视，意在丹田，气行督任二脉（图 15-3）。

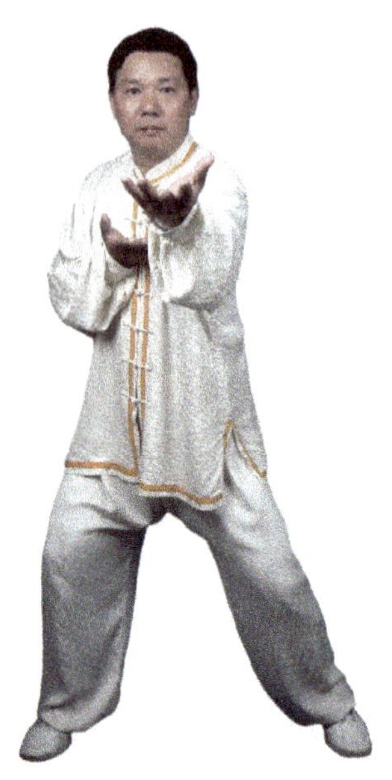

图 15-4 蛇盘左势

3）蛇盘左势

上动略停，体微向左转，身体重心向上升起，面向南方自然站立，提踵。两臂外旋，双手由脐下向上、向左前方弧形上托。左掌在前上方，与肩同高，掌心向上，指尖向前；右掌指斜指左肘关节内侧，掌心向上。与之同时，丹田向内凹、吸气。舌顶上腭，牙齿轻扣。目随左掌移动，意在涌泉穴上提（图 15-4）。

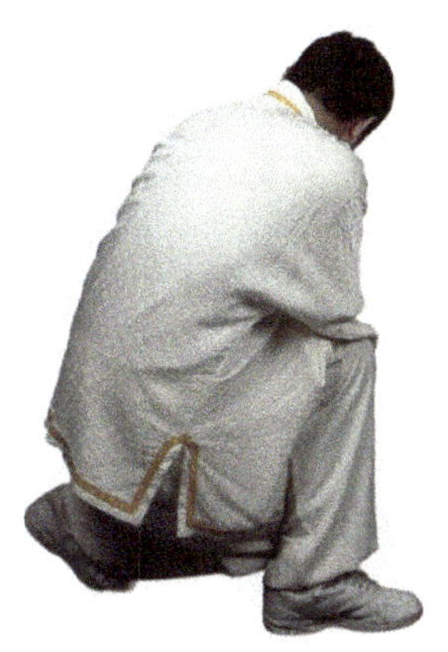

图 15-5 蛇盘左势

上动不停，体向左转，两腿交叉的同时向下蹲，左脚全脚着地并向外展，右脚跟离地，重心偏于左腿成左蛇盘步。同时，两臂内旋，左手掌回挂停于胸前，掌指向上，掌心向右；右手掌下插至右脚跟上方，掌指斜指右脚跟，掌心向右小腿。同时，丹田向外凸、呼气。舌守下腭，牙齿微扣。目随身移，意在肾俞穴，气行足太阳膀胱经（图 15-5）。

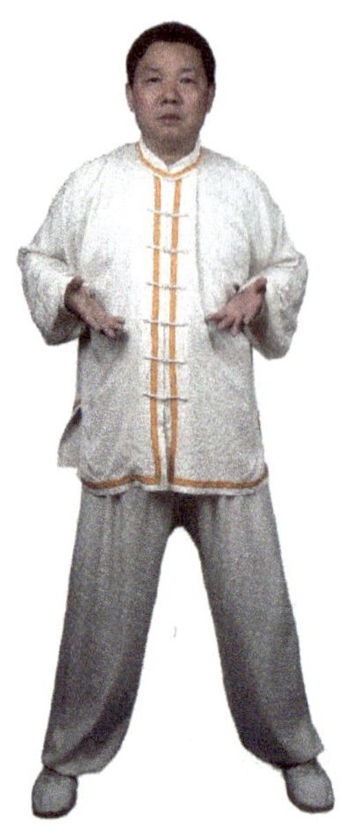

图 15-6 右转小收

4）右转小收

上动略停，调整 2 次呼吸后，身体重心升起，体向右转，仍面向南方。两臂外旋，两手随之向内上抬，掌根部停靠于两乳下。双手指尖向前，掌心向上。与之同时，丹田向内凹、吸气。舌顶上腭，牙齿轻扣，目视前方（图 15-6）。

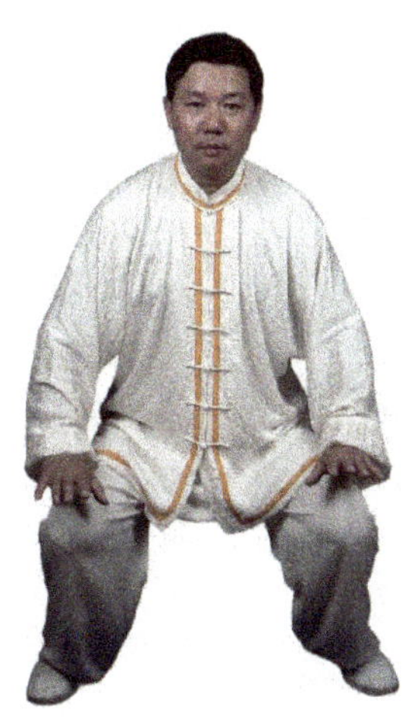

图 15-7 右转小收

上动不停，身体重心下降，两腿屈膝下蹲成马步。同时，两臂内旋，两肘合抱，手向体前弧形下按，停于腹前。掌心向下，指尖向前方。同时，丹田向外凸、呼气。舌守下腭，牙齿微扣。目微下视，意在丹田，气行督任二脉（图 15-7、15-8）。

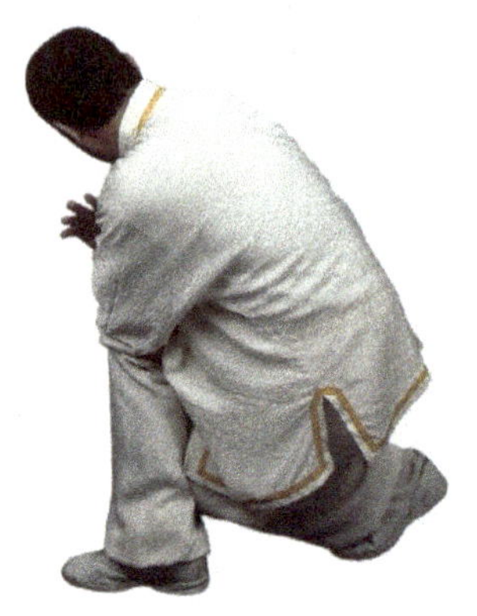

图 15-8 蛇盘右势

5）蛇盘右势

动作方法完全同蛇盘左势，惟左右方向相反（参阅图 15-4、15-5）。

6）化气养身

动作方法完全同推山功无极初开（参阅图 2-2）。 上动不停，动作方法完全同无极功混元一气（参阅图 1-8）。

武当气功

要领与功能：

练习蛇盘功，掌向下的插劲，要与另外手掌，向上的穿劲合在一齐。两臂要紧抱，髋要松，肛要提，肩要扣，肘要坠，头要向上顶。以腰带动全身的转动，并与两腿屈膝交叉下蹲的动作同时合拍，整齐一致。

蛇盘功主要练习腰部的灵活性，气行大周天。腰部和脊椎部在整个运动中，起到主宰作用，要始终保持正直。因动作的需要，可以收缩、摇晃、屈曲，以助内气运行。全身上下，好象拧绳一样，快速中带有一种弹力。摇膀活髋，全身辗转。气行大周天，就是武当气功“练气化神”的过程。它是在练习小周天的基础上进行的，通过内气运行习练，使神和气，和劲力更加密切的结合，相抱不离。内气循环的路线，除了循行督脉、任脉小周天外，又可以在其它经络流动。

练习武当气功，不可自专自用，而固执不通。身外形式，要顺遂自然无形中自增气力。身体内中要中和元贯，无形中自增灵气。意念要求松静自然，意气相随、炼养结合、吸气绵绵、呼气微微。最后达到呼吸、意念、神气自然随合。

练习方法：

每次练习以 6 次或 12 次为一组，可以反复练习。动作的幅度大小、高低不限，以个人的年龄、力量大小、体质强弱而定。

武当气功

点穴

督脉 GV[who]

任脉 CV[who]

涌泉穴 KC-1[who]

肾俞穴 BL-23[who]

足太阳膀胱经 BL[who]

第十六节　白蛇吐芯功

白蛇吐芯气内守，
用功用意摇摆头。
滔滔江河归大海，
以静待动妙悠悠。

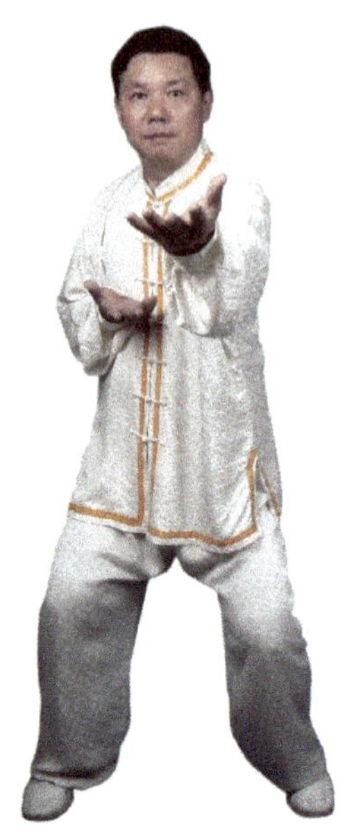

图 16-1 白蛇吐芯左势

1）预备势

动作方法完全同无极功预备势（参阅图 1-1、1-2、1-3、1-4）。

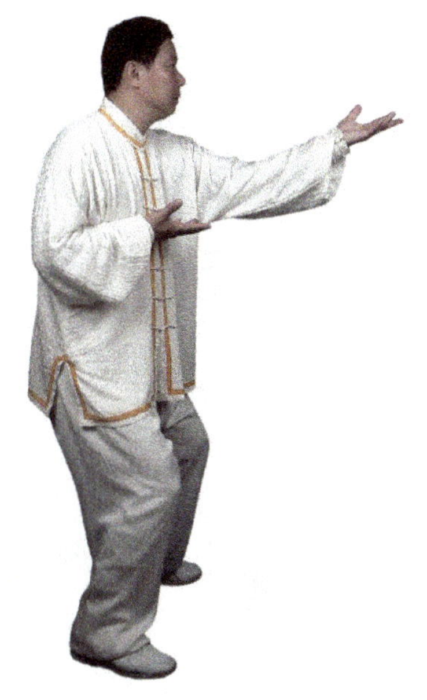

图 16-2 白蛇吐芯左势

2）白蛇吐芯左势

上动略停，体微向左转，两臂外旋，掌由体侧前向左前上方弧形托起。左掌在前与鼻同高，掌心向上，指尖向前；右掌停于左肩前，指尖向前，掌心向上。同时，丹田向内凹、吸气。舌顶上腭，牙齿轻扣。目视左掌，意在手心劳宫穴、头顶心百会穴、脚心涌泉，3 心吸上、中、下 3 气（图 16-1、16-2）。

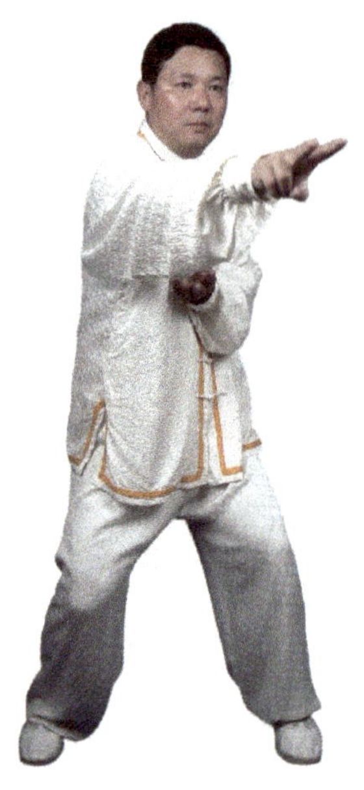

图 16-3 白蛇吐芯左势

上动不停，体微向右转，身体重心下降，两腿屈膝下蹲成马步。同时，两掌食指、中指伸直分开，其余 3 指屈于手心，拇指压在无名指和小指的第一指骨节上。右掌由右胸部向前上方翻转戳出，与鼻同高，指尖向前，掌心向下；左掌随之而动向内回，停于左乳下，指尖向前，掌心向上。与之同时，丹田向外凸、缓缓呼气。舌守下腭，牙齿微扣。目视右手指，意在扭腰拉掌（图 16-3）。

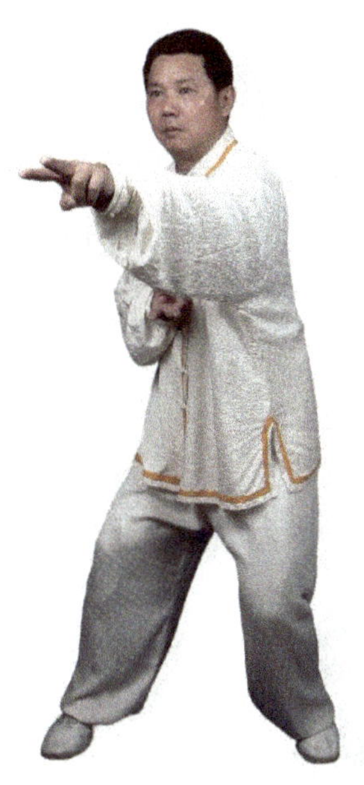

图 16-4 白蛇吐芯左势

紧接上动不停，体微向右转，双手指型不变。左臂上抬前伸，左掌由胸左侧向前戳出，与鼻同高，指尖向前，掌心向下；右臂下压，右掌随之转动回收，停于右胸下，指尖向前，掌心向上。与之同时，丹田继续向外凸、缓缓呼气。舌守下腭，牙齿微扣。目视左掌指尖，意在丹田（图 16-4）。

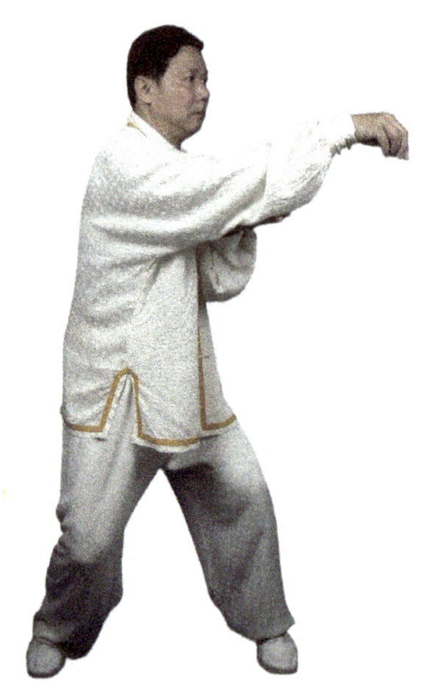

图 16-5 以静待动

3）以静待动

上动略停，体微向左转，两腿屈膝下蹲成马步。右臂内旋，右手 5 指并拢成蛇头掌，由胸前翻转而出，屈肘停于头前；左臂外旋，左手随之而动，回收停于右肘下，指尖向前，掌心向上。与之同时，丹田向内凹、吸气。舌顶上腭，牙齿微扣。目视右蛇头掌，意在肘尖沉坠，气行手三阳经（图 16-5）。

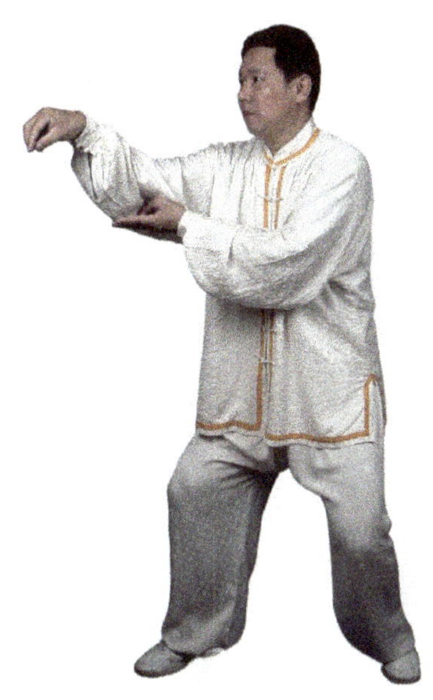

图 16-6 以静待动

上动不停，体向右转，腰部晃动上肢手势不变，随身转动。同时，丹田向外凸、呼气。舌守下腭，牙齿微扣。目随右蛇头掌移动，意在心静待动（图 16-6）。

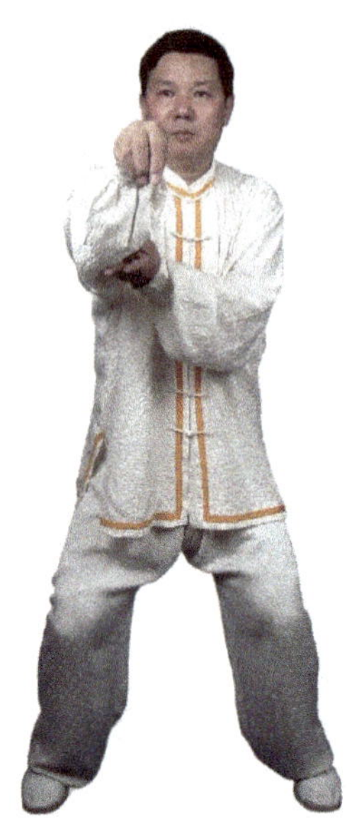

图 16-7 以静待动

上动不停，身体晃动向左转，两腿逐渐伸直。重心随转体升起，面向南方，自然站立。上体动作姿势不变。与之同时，丹田向内凹、吸气。舌顶上腭，牙齿轻扣。目随右掌移动，意在肾俞穴，气行带脉（图 16-7）。

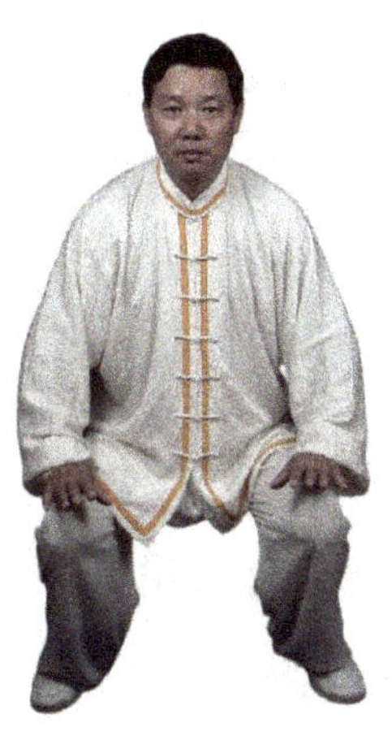

图 16-8 以静待动

上动略停，两腿屈膝下蹲成马步。同时，两臂内旋，两肘合抱，手向体前弧形下按，停于腹前。掌心向下，指尖向前。与之同时，丹田向外凸、呼气。舌守下腭，牙齿微扣。目微下视，意在丹田，气行督任二脉（图 16-8）。

4）白蛇吐芯右势

动作方法完全同白蛇吐芯左势，惟左右方向相反（参阅图 16-1、16-2、16-3、16-4）。

5）内守还原

动作方法完全同推山功无极初开（参阅图 2-1）。上动不停，动作方法完全同无极功混元一气（参阅图 1-8）。

武当气功

要领与功能：

练习白蛇吐芯功，2 指向前的戳劲，要与前手向回的拉劲同步，如拉弓一般。周身务必放松，稍微含胸，立身中正。精神集中，以腰带动全身一齐抖动，重心的下落与腰部的晃动要同时进行，转身时要含胸、提踵，松肩、坠肘、提肛拔顶。

练习本功法还应要做到：3 心要並、3 意要连、4 梢要齐。3 心要並者，头顶心百会穴向下凹、脚心涌泉穴向上提、手心劳宫穴向回缩，使 3 气会聚于丹田。顶心不向下，则上气不能入丹田；脚心不上提，则下气不能收于丹田；手心不向回收，则外气不能缩于丹田。因此，必须 3 心合並，气才能归聚于一处炼丹。

3 意要连者，即心意、气意、力意，连贯如一。此 3 意，以心为谋士、以气为元帅、以力为将士。气不充盈，则力不从心，虽有谋也无所用。因此，气、意先炼好，才能向外统帅力意，向内统帅和应心意。

4 梢要齐者，即舌顶、齿扣、手指、脚趾扣、毛孔要紧。舌顶上腭，则津液上注气血流通，舌守下腭，津液随呼气归于丹田；齿扣，气可以贯注于骨髓；手指、脚趾内扣，气可以行之于筋；毛孔紧。没有先后、迟速之分，如果四项之中有一项做不到，则易发生气散、力怠、精神不振的现象。

动作中的提踵，是让炼功者渐渐达到踵息之境界。庄子曰："真人之息以踵，众人之息以喉。"一般常人呼吸，都是随咽喉而下的，至胸下中脘穴处而回，不能与元气相连，象鱼儿饮水口进腮出一般。即庄子所谓“真人之息以踵”，踵者，真息深深之意。可以说平常人之息是后天气之呼吸，真人之息乃先天气，即潜气之运行，其息可以直达足跟。丹经云：“顶门之核露堂堂，脚跟之机活泼泼”。在炼功中，运用细小微微的意念活动，来调整呼吸，排除杂念。还要把这种思维活动，逐渐降低到最微限度，以至消失。脑子里空空静静，以任真气在全身循行，上至头顶百会，下至脚尖、脚跟。重心升降和提踵，可以调动足 3 阴经、足 3 阳经，对肝、脾、肾经也有一定的作用。同时，提踵也可以使全身最大限度地拉长，因而，对强腰健肾也起到了好的作用。

练习方法：

每次练习以 6 次或 12 次为一组，可以反复练习。动作的幅度大小、高低不限，以个人的年龄大、力量大小、体质强弱而定。

点穴

劳宫穴 PC-8[who]
百会穴 GV-20[who]
涌泉穴 KC-1[who]
肾俞穴 BL-23[who]
带脉 GIV, GB-26[who]
督脉 GV[who]
任脉 CV[who]
中脘穴 CV-12[who]

第十七节 狸猫上树功

狸猫上树气沟通，
表里上下劲无穷。
漫云肾气生人体，
还要后天精气充。

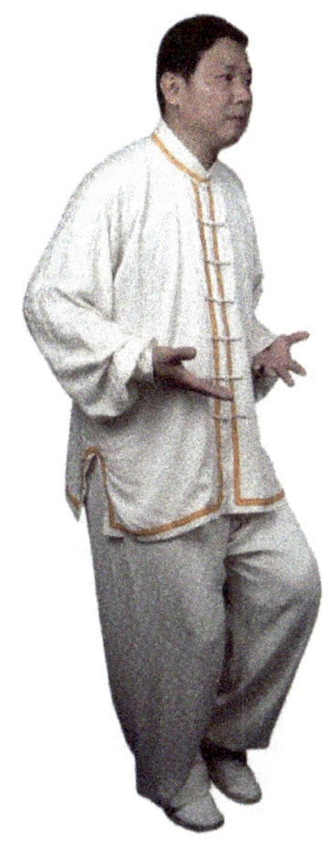

图 17-1 狸猫上树左势

1）预备势

动作方法完全同无极功预备势（参阅图 1-1、1-2、1-3、1-4）。

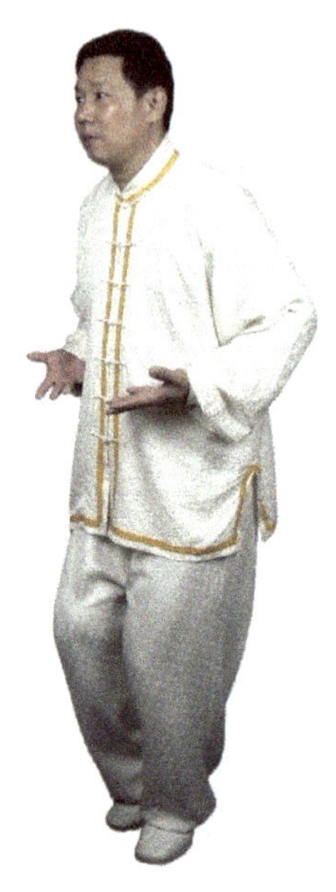

图 17-2 狸猫上树左势

2）狸猫上树左势

上动略停，体向左转 45 度，重心移至右腿上，微向下蹲。左脚脚跟提起，脚面绷直，脚尖稍向内扣，并虚点地面成左高虚步。两臂外旋，双手由体侧弧形上捧，阳掌停于胸前侧。指尖向前，掌心向上。同时，丹田向内凹、吸气。舌顶上腭，牙齿轻扣。目随身移，意在提脚心涌泉穴（图 17-1、17-2）。

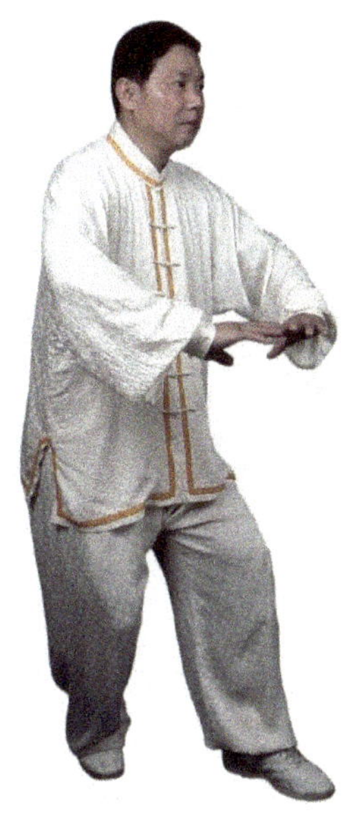

图 17-3 狸猫上树左势

上动不停，身体重心下移，左脚全脚掌着地成左四六步，两臂内旋，双手由胸前翻转下按，与腹同高，指尖向前，掌下向下。同时，丹田向外凸、呼气。舌守下腭，牙齿微扣。目视前下方，意在脊端，劲由脊发（图 17-3）。

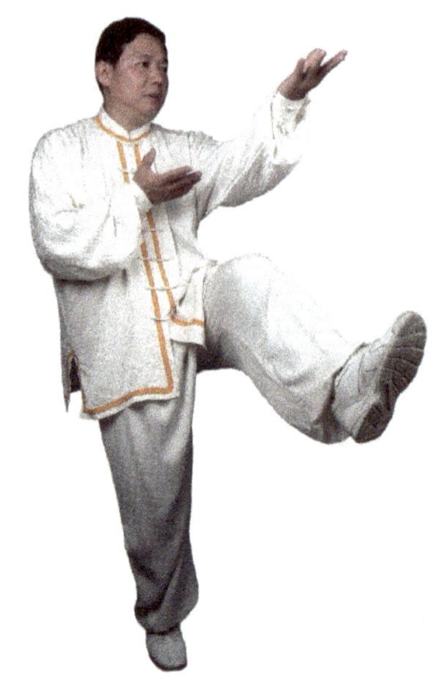

图 17-4 狸猫上树左势

上动略停，身体重心后移于右腿上；左脚尖外摆提起，向前蹬出略高于膝部，脚尖向左上方，脚心向前成狸猫左起势。同时，两臂外旋，双手向前上方穿刺，左手在前上方，与喉同高；右手在左肘关节处。双手指尖向前，掌心向上。与之同时，丹田向内凹、吸气。舌顶上腭，牙齿轻扣。目视左前方，意在左脚尖处侠溪穴，气行足少阳胆经（图 17-4）。

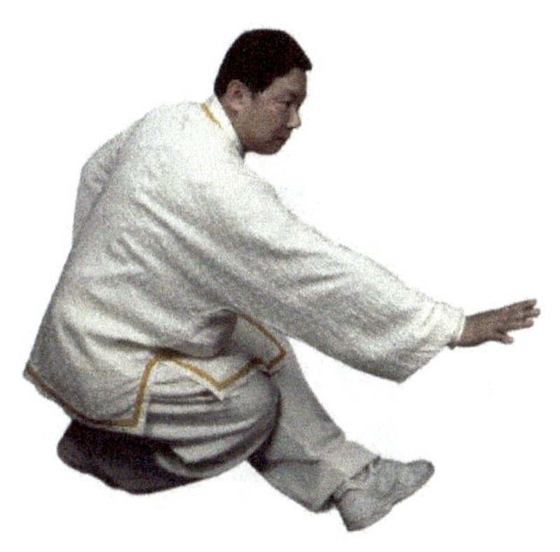

图 17-5 狸猫上树左势

紧接上动不停，身体重心下落，左脚尖外摆向前下方踩；右脚跟离地，身体微向前倾，臀部坐于右小腿上成狸猫左落势。同时，双臂内旋，两手一齐用力向前下方劈斩按压。左手落于左大腿上侧，指尖向前，掌心向下；右手低于脐部，停于左脚上方，指尖向前上方，掌心向前下方。与之同时，丹田向外凸、呼气。舌守下腭，牙齿微扣。目视前下，意在大腿（图 17-5）。

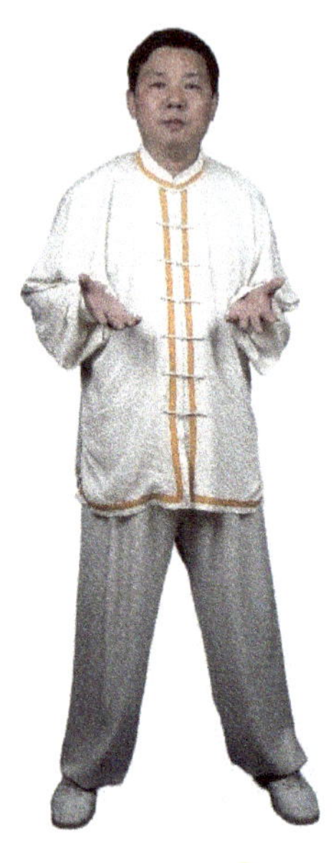

图 17-6 转身小收

3）转身小收

上动略停，身体右转 45 度。调整 2 次呼吸后，两腿伸直，面南自然站立。与之同时，两臂外旋，两手随之向内上抬，掌根部停靠于两乳下。指尖向前，掌心向上。与之同时，丹田向内凹、吸气。舌顶上腭，牙齿轻扣，目视前方（图 17-6）。

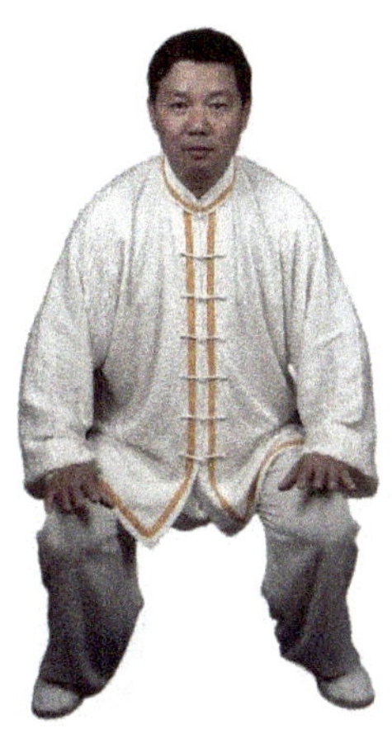

图 17-7 转身小收

上动不停，身体重心下降，两腿屈膝下蹲成马步。同时，两臂内旋，两肘合抱，手向体前弧形下按，停于腹前。掌心向下，指尖向前方。同时，丹田向外凸、呼气。舌守下腭，牙齿微扣。目微下视，意在丹田，气行督任二脉（图 17-7、17-8）。

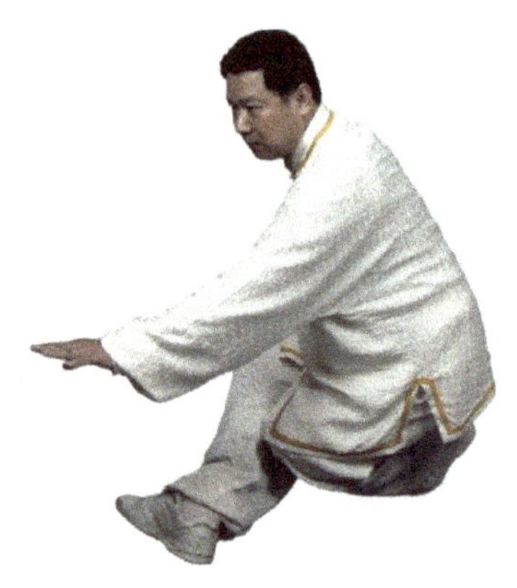

图 17-8 转身小收

4）狸猫上树右势

动作方法完全同狸猫上树左势，惟左右方向相反（参阅图 17-1、17-2、17-3、17-4、17-5）。

5）收势还原

动作方法完全同推山功无极初开（参阅图 2-1）。上动不停，动作方法完全同无极功混元一气（参阅图 1-8）。

武当气功

要领与功能：

狸猫上树功的蹬腿动作，要于两掌向上穿刺同时，脚、掌一齐到，落势时鼻、脚、指 3 尖要相对，在一个垂直面上。身体重心分为前 3 分、后 7 分。前脚要尽量伸直，臀部要接近后脚跟。腰要塌，头要上顶，后膝要顶着前腿膝关节后面。舌要上顶、下守调气，齿要轻扣、微扣，使气血循行全身经络穴位。精神务必集中，以腰带动身体一齐转动。肘不离肋，手不离心，钻、劈、进身，都要合拍齐全。

人以气为本，以心为根，以息为主。一呼百脉皆开，一吸百脉皆合。天地万物的旋转运行，都不出呼吸 2 字。呼吸的方法有 3 节道理和 3 步功夫，即练习中国武当气功之准绳。1 节，呼吸自然任意，有形于外，称之谓调息，也叫做炼精化气第 1 步功夫；2 节，呼吸有形于内，着意于丹田之呼吸，称之谓息调，又名曰"胎息"，也叫做炼气化神第 2 步功夫；3 节，心肾相交的内呼吸，无形无象，绵绵若存，似有非有，无声无息，也谓之炼神还虚第 3 步功夫。

调气法总的要求是：轻出、缓入，呼吸以鼻，切忌用口（鼻子不通气者除外）。最初积蓄真意与气息，以致满足。中立而不倚，和而不流，无形无相。

练功中意念上要做到 3 守： 1 守清、 2 守盈、 3 守窍。守清，就是守清则自明，知公则心平，神清意平，乃能制物之情；守盈，就是天之道损有余，奉不足，故不能，行强梁之努气，以求长生久视；守窍，就是将真意固守规矩中一窍，则可以逐渐收伏其心以至于入定，定则真阳自发，意气自生。久之神气融合，神胎自结。

武当气功

练习方法：

每次练习以 6 次或 12 次为一组，可以反复练习。动作的幅度大小高低不限，以个人的年龄、力量大小、体质强弱而定。

点穴

督脉 GV[who]
任脉 CV[who]
涌泉穴 KC-1[who]
侠溪穴 GB-43[who]
足少阳胆经 GB[who]

第十八节　群峰朝顶功

七十二峰拜金顶，
三十六崖力补坤。
丹田炼成长生宝，
万两黄金不与人。

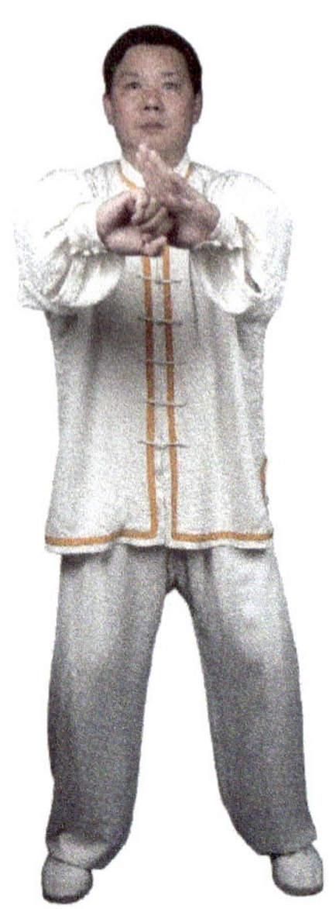

图 18-1 诚心拜山

1）预备势

动作方法完全同无极功预备势（参阅图 1-1、1-2、1-3、1-4）。

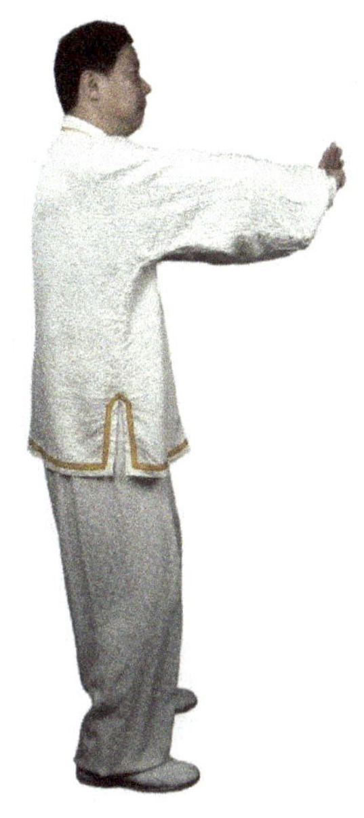

图 18-2 诚心拜山

2）诚心拜山

上动略停，两臂外旋，双手由体侧向上抄起，停于唇下承浆穴处，左掌指尖向上，掌心向右；右掌变拳，倚着左掌心劳宫穴，拳面向上，拳心向左。同时，丹田向内凹、吸气。舌顶上腭，牙齿轻扣。目微闭合，意在头顶百会穴（图 18-1、18-2）。

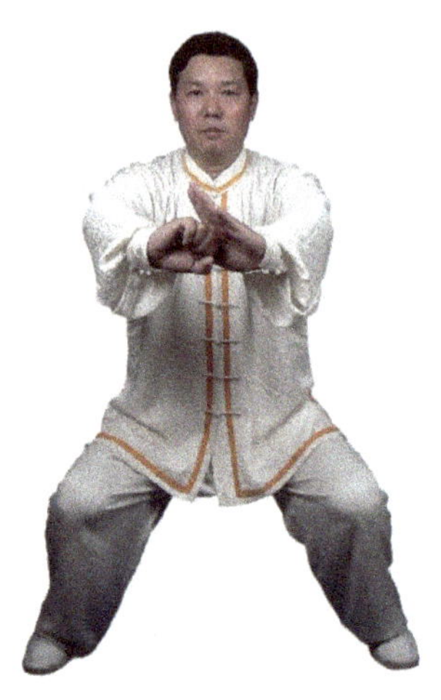

图 18-3 诚心拜山

上动不停，两腿屈膝下蹲，身体前俯。两膝关节内扣，提踵，肘关节相抱。双手手型不变，随之而动弧形下落。与之同时，丹田向外凸、呼气。舌守下腭，牙齿微扣。目向内视，意在丹田（图 18-3）。

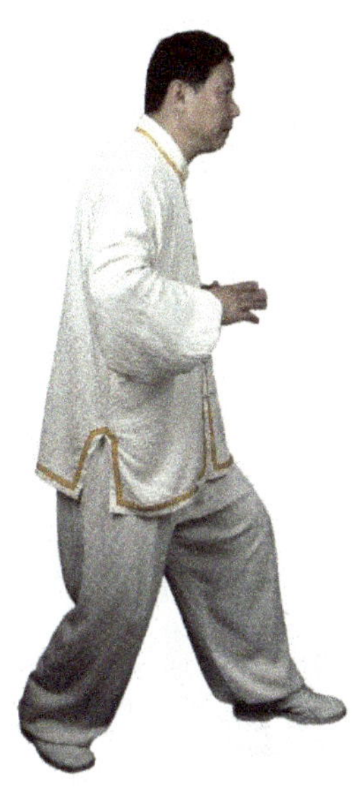

图 18-4 群峰朝顶左势

3）群峰朝顶左势

上动略停，体向左转 90 度，重心上升右脚尖内扣屈膝微蹲，左脚跟离地，脚面绷平，脚尖稍内扣并虚点地面，左膝微屈，重心落于右腿成左高虚步。同时，两臂内旋，双手由头前向下划弧反撑，停于腹前。指尖相对，掌心斜向前下方。同时，丹田向内凹、吸气。舌顶上腭，牙齿轻扣。目随身转，意在沉肩坠肘，气行手少阳三焦经（图 18-4）。

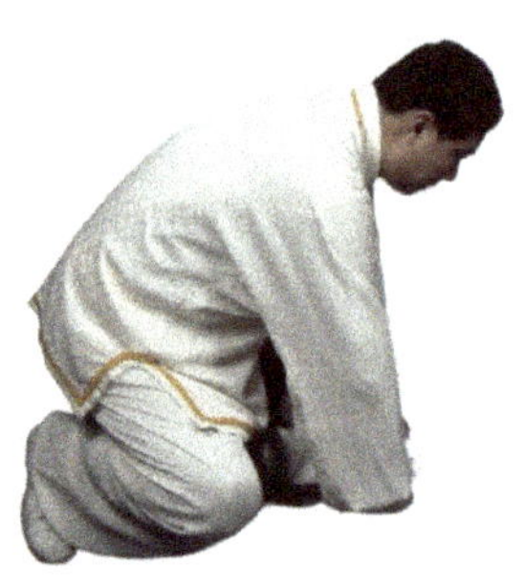

图 18-5 群峰朝顶左势

上动不停，身体重心前移，落于左腿上；右脚尖着地，提踵。两腿屈膝全蹲，上体压在左腿上。两掌向前下按压，停于左脚尖前，指尖相对，掌心向下按地。与之同时，丹田向外凸、呼气。舌守下腭牙齿微扣。目视前下方，意在提右踵，气行足太阳膀胱经（图 18-5）。

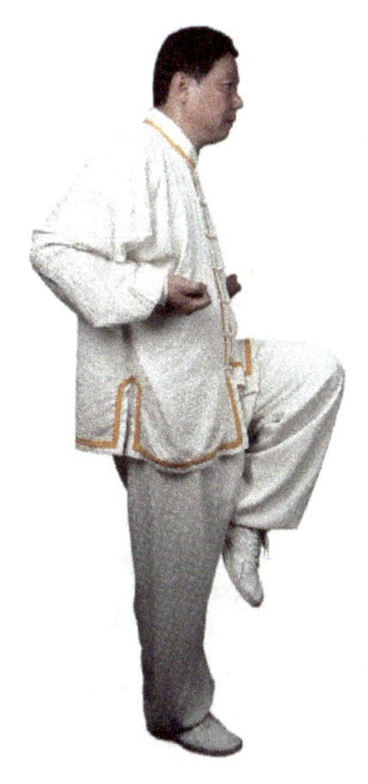

图 18-6 群峰朝顶左势

上动略停，身体重心移于右腿上，右腿伸直，右脚全脚着地；左腿屈提，脚尖向下，脚面绷直成左独立势。同时，两臂外旋，两掌在体前划弧，停于丹田两侧。掌心向前，指尖向下。同时，丹田向内凹、吸气。舌顶上腭，牙齿轻扣。目视前方，意在 10 指抓捏，气行手三阳经（图 18-6）。

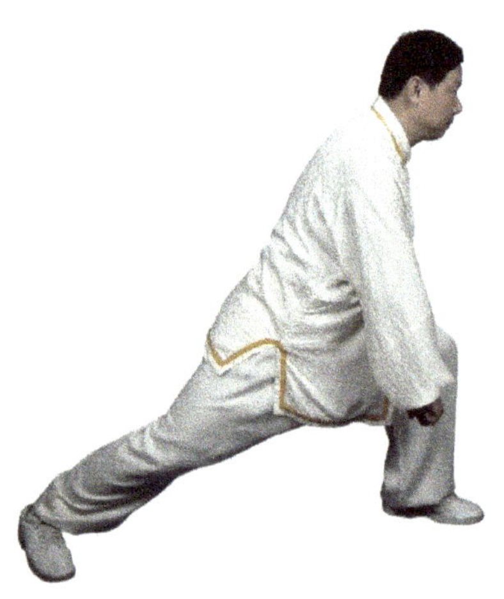

图 18-7 群峰朝顶左势

紧接上动不停，左脚向前下落，脚尖微向内扣，屈膝半蹲；右腿挺膝伸直，脚尖内扣成左弓步。同时两臂内旋，双手屈曲抓握成拳向下砸落，停于左膝关节前下两侧。两拳相距 10 厘米，拳心向内，拳面向下。下砸同时，丹田向外凸、呼气。舌守下腭，牙齿微扣。目从两拳之间下视，意在伸肘催气（图 18-7）。

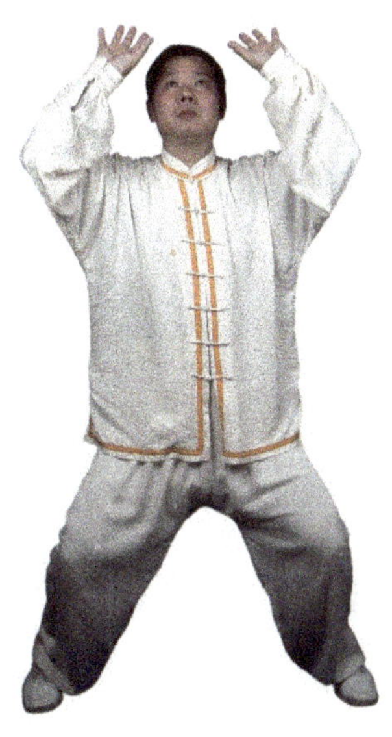

图 18-8 俯身按掌

4）俯身按掌

上动略停，体向右转 90 度。身体重心随之升起，成面向南方自然站立势。同时，两臂屈肘上抬，两拳变掌，以手背领气弧形托捧，停于头前。指尖向上，掌心向前。托捧同时，丹田向内凹、吸气。舌守下腭，牙齿轻扣。目视前上意在小指少冲穴翻转，气行手少阴心经（图 18-8）。

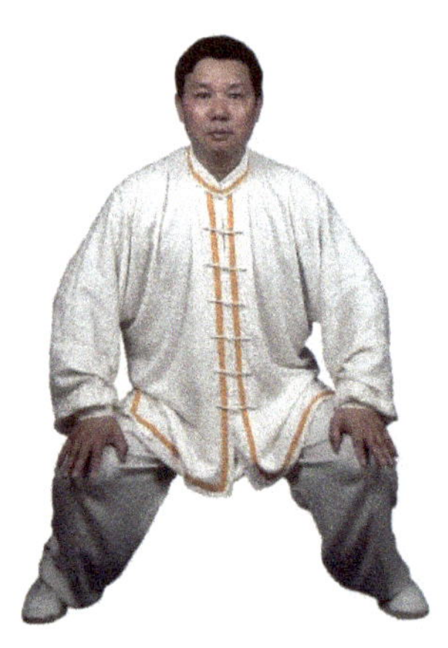

图 18-9 俯身按掌

上动不停，两腿屈蹲成马步。上体前倾，两掌由头前弧形下压，停于膝关节前。掌根靠在髌骨上，指尖向下斜指脚尖。下压同时，丹田向外凸、呼气。舌守下腭，牙齿微扣。目视前下方，意在丹田，气行大周天（图 18-9）。

5）群峰朝顶右势

动作方法完全同群峰朝顶左势，惟左右方向相反（参阅图 18-4、18-5、18-6、18-7）。

6） 练功归原

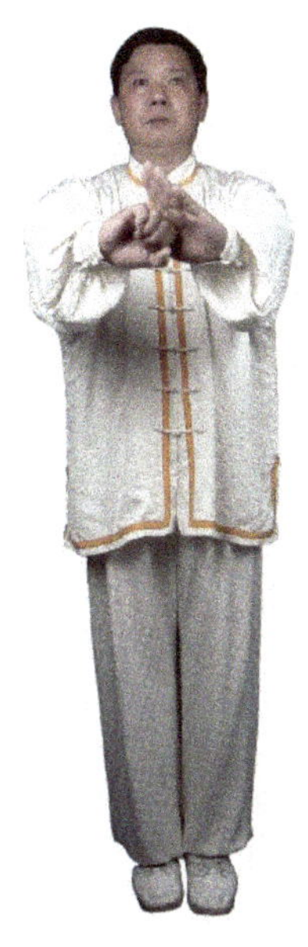

图 18-10 练功归原

上动略停，体左转、面向南方。两臂向外旋，双手由体侧向上抄起，停于唇下承桨处，左掌指尖向上掌心向右；右掌变拳倚着左掌心劳宫穴，拳面向上，拳心向左。与之同时，丹田向内凹、吸气。舌顶上腭，牙齿轻扣。目微闭合，意在头顶百会穴。而后，两手下落成立正姿势（图 18-10）。

武当气功

要领与功能：

练功中，脚的上步、垫步、提起、下落都要与手的运行、阴掌、阳掌、划弧、绕环等动作配合一致，并要以腰为运动的主宰，向上带动脊背、肩、肘、手、指，向下带动髋、膝、足、趾。所谓：“一枝动，百枝摇”就是这个道理。群峰朝顶功上一种以呼吸为主，辅以导引、按摩的养生内壮功夫。

先哲修炼，重视气对人体的作用，认为至天地至万物，无不需要气，赖以生存。故曰：“气聚则生，气散则亡”。人欲长寿者，必须要爱气、养气、尊神意、重精。善于练功行气之人，内可以壮体，外可以祛恶抗邪。行气之时，要求凝神净虑，专气致柔，呼吸吐纳，做到：轻、缓、匀、长、深。

轻，呼吸轻细；
缓，进出气舒缓；
匀，呼吸节拍匀致；
长，呼吸间隔时间长；
深，气深入肺腑百脉，通融全身。

炼丹之道，源于古代方术。原指在炉鼎中烧炼矿石药物，以制造“长生不老”的灵丹妙药。后来，被道家们称谓炼“外丹”。而后，又将人体拟作炉鼎，以炼养身体内的精、气、神，作为修炼内丹的药物。古人云；“上药三品，神、气与精，恍恍惚惚杳杳冥冥”。精、气、神，虽然并称为炼内丹之药，但是，排列顺序不同。

武当气功

“神”为君是主，“精、气”为臣是客。万神为一神，万气为一气，以一而生万，摄万而归于一，皆生之我“神”。所以，要求在武当气功，全部功法练习过程中，皆以“神”领气，以“神”炼精，始终不离开“神”字，既是“神”为主宰，“气”为动力，“精”为基础。这 3 种人体生命之中的 3 大元素，互向为用。古人云：“心虚则神凝，神凝则气聚，气聚则精生。”然后，通过功法养炼互换合化的过程，逐步成为返老还童的物资基础。张真人在《悟真篇》说：“人人本有长生药，自是迷徒狂摆抛。甘露降时、天地合，黄芽生处、坎离交。井蛙应谓无龙窟，篱雀安知有风巢。丹熟自然金满屋，何须寻草学烧茅？”就是指人人自己身中都有长生的丹药，可惜不懂得珍惜而白白地抛掉了。阴阳相合、精神合炼，人体生命代谢之元素可以新生。“甘露”既是指先天一气，从泥丸下降至丹田中“黄芽”上下交会，凝聚成“圣胎”，称谓丹熟。“金满屋”则是指：练功者已达到精、气，神三花聚顶，心、肝、脾、肺、肾五气朝元之境界。

练习方法：

每次练习以 6 次或 12 次为一组，可以反复练习。动作的幅度大小高低不限，以个人的年龄、力量大小、体质强弱而定。

武当气功

点穴

承浆穴 CV-24[who]

劳宫穴 PC-8[who]

百会穴 GV-20[who]

手少阳三焦经 TB[who]

足太阳膀胱经 BL[who]

少冲穴 HT-9[who]

手少阴心经 HT[who]

武当气功

点穴目录

第一节　无极功

劳宫穴 PC-8[who]

涌泉穴 KC-1[who]

膻中穴 Chest Center CV-17[who]

厥阴肝经

玄关窍

百会穴 GV-20[who]

气海 CV-6[who]

第二节　推山功

真元

元气

督脉 GV[who]

任脉 CV[who]

会阴 CV-1[who]

第二节　雁飞功

章门穴 LV-13

劳宫穴 PC-8[who]

玄关窍

督脉 GV[who]

百会穴 s GV-20[who]

曲池穴 LI-11[who]

涌泉穴 KC-1[who]

第四节　鹤拗功

劳宫穴 PC-8[who]

三里 ST-36

内关 PC-6[who]

外关TB-5

中冲 PC-9[who]

厥阴心包经 PC^{who}
百会穴 GV-20^{who}

第五节 托天功

督脉 GV^{who}
任脉 CV^{who}
神封穴 KI-23^{who}
劳宫穴 PC-8^{who}
玄关窍）
神庭穴 GV-24^{who}
华盖CV-20^{who}
少泽 SI-1^{who}
太阳小肠经 I
涌泉穴 KC-1^{who}
百会穴 GV-20^{who}
尾闾关
辘轳关
玉枕 BK-9^{who}
膻中

第六节 两仪功

督脉 GV^{who}
任脉 CV^{who}
期门 LV-14
涌泉穴KC-1^{who}
劳宫穴 PC-8^{who}
手太阴肺经 LU^{who}
会阴 CV-1^{who}
鹊桥
尾闾关
腰阳关 GV-3^{who}
命门穴 GV-4^{who}

阴交 CV-7[who]

气海 CV-6[who]

第七节　四象功

督脉 GV[who]

任脉CV[who]

冲脉 PV

百会穴 GV-20[who]

涌泉穴 KC-1[who]

劳宫穴 PC-8[who]

第八节　棚捋功

督脉GV[who]

任脉 CV[who]

劳宫穴 PC-8[who]

涌泉穴 KC-1[who]

手阳明大肠经 LI[who]

水道穴 ST-28[who]

足阳明胃经 [who]

商阳穴 LI-1[who]

带脉 GIV, GB-26[who]

冲脉 PV

第九节　琵琶功

督脉 GV[who]

任脉 CV[who]

劳宫穴PC-8[who]

百会穴 GV-20[who]

四白穴 ST-2[who]

气海 CV-6[who]

第十节　抖翎功

督脉 GV[who]

任脉 CV[who]
百会穴 GV-20[who]
少冲穴 HT-9[who]
劳宫穴 PC-8[who]
脉门 HT-9[who]
涌泉穴KC-1[who]

第十一节　白猿献果功

劳宫穴 PC-8[who]
带脉 GB-26[who]
足少阳胆经 GB[who]
承浆穴 CV-24[who]
涌泉穴 KC-1[who]
手太阴肺经 LU[who]
厥阴心包经 PC [who]
玉堂穴CV-18[who]
玄关窍

第十二节　丹凤朝阳功

内关PC-6[who]
大陵穴 PC-7[who]
周荣穴 SP-20[who]
百会穴 GV-20[who]
太阴脾经 SP[who]
外关 TB-5
大陵穴PC-7[who]
周荣穴SP-20[who]
太阴脾经 SP[who]
劳宫穴 PC-8[who]
会阴 CV-1[who]
涌泉穴 KC-1[who]
命门穴 GV-4[who]

夹脊穴
玉枕 BK-9[who]
风府穴 GV-16[who]
人中穴 GV-26[who]
承浆穴 CV-24[who]
任脉 CV[who]
长强穴 GV-1[who]

第十三节　拨草寻蛇功

劳宫穴 PC-8[who]
极泉穴 HT-1[who]
百会穴 GV-20[who]
孔最 LU-6[who]
手太阴肺经 LU[who]
神门穴 HT-7[who]
手阳明大肠经 LI[who]
督脉 GV[who]
任脉 CV[who]

第十四节　龙虎相交功

督脉 GV[who]
任脉CV[who]
中庭穴 CV-16[who]
商阳穴 LI-1[who]
手阳明大肠经 LI[who]
承浆穴 CV-24[who]
人中穴GV-26[who]
玄关窍

第十五节　蛇盘功

督脉 GV[who]
任脉 CV[who]
涌泉穴 KC-1[who]

肾俞穴 BL-23[who]

足太阳膀胱经 BL[who]

第十六节　白蛇吐芯功

劳宫穴 PC-8[who]

百会穴 GV-20[who]

涌泉穴 KC-1[who]

肾俞穴 BL-23[who]

带脉 GIV, GB-26[who]

督脉 GV[who]

任脉 CV[who]

中脘穴 CV-12[who]

第十七节　狸猫上树功

督脉 GV[who]

任脉 CV[who]

涌泉穴 KC-1[who]

侠溪穴 GB-43[who]

足少阳胆经 GB[who]

第十八节　群峰朝顶功

承浆穴 CV-24[who]

劳宫穴 PC-8[who]

百会穴 GV-20[who]

手少阳三焦经 TB[who]

足太阳膀胱经 BL[who]

少冲穴 HT-9[who]

手少阴心经 HT[who]

图目录

武当气功

关于作者：刘玉增 1958 年 6 岁时开始跟随祖父刘文周$习少林武术。12 岁时继承师父王希孝传授 武当内家拳戈。刘玉增是 31 代少林寺弟子， 也是现代中国嵩山少林寺武术名人之一，1999 " 年列入《国际杰出名人绿》。独自编著出 普玉 I3 本武术专著，有 100 余篇论文论著在 国家级公开杂志上铋表。刘教授居住工作在 中国古代殷商的首都域市一河南省郑州市。

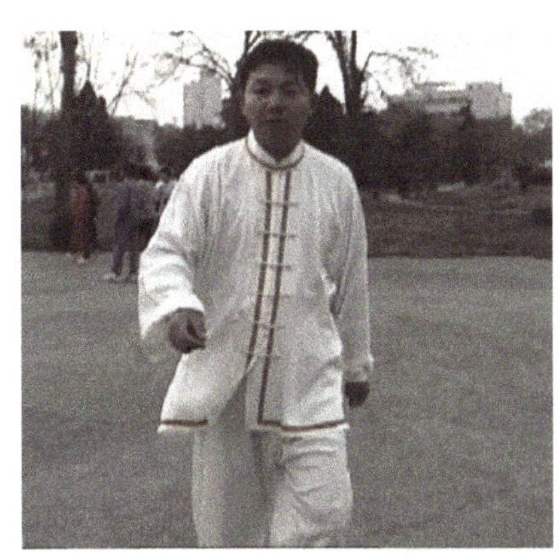

刘玉增这人民公园，郑州市。1999

译者简介：特丽。摩根于 1985 年开始跟随黄伟伦学习杨式太极拳。1989 年，她在休斯敦举行的全美锦标赛上获得第一名。1990 年，她前往中国教英语。 在那里，她认识了刘玉增教授，并开始向他学习武当内拳、形意、八卦、剑法。 摩根女士出生于堪萨斯城，在 UMKC 获得英语学士学位。 1995 年，她被列入世界女性名人录。 她的大部分职业生涯都在技术领域工作，撰写了数十篇软件手册和技术文章。 摩根女士开发并维护了武当研究会、公司网站和公司出版物。

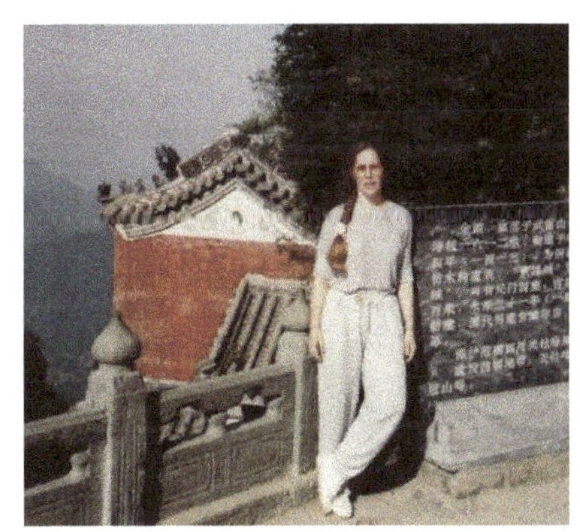

特丽摩根这武当山，1995

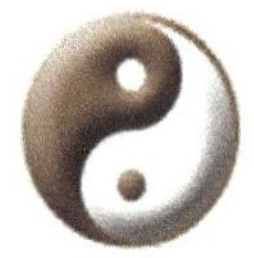

武当研究会

www.ingramcontent.com/pod-product-compliance
Lightning Source LLC
Chambersburg PA
CBHW060018030426
42334CB00019B/2084

* 9 7 8 0 9 6 7 2 8 8 9 8 7 *